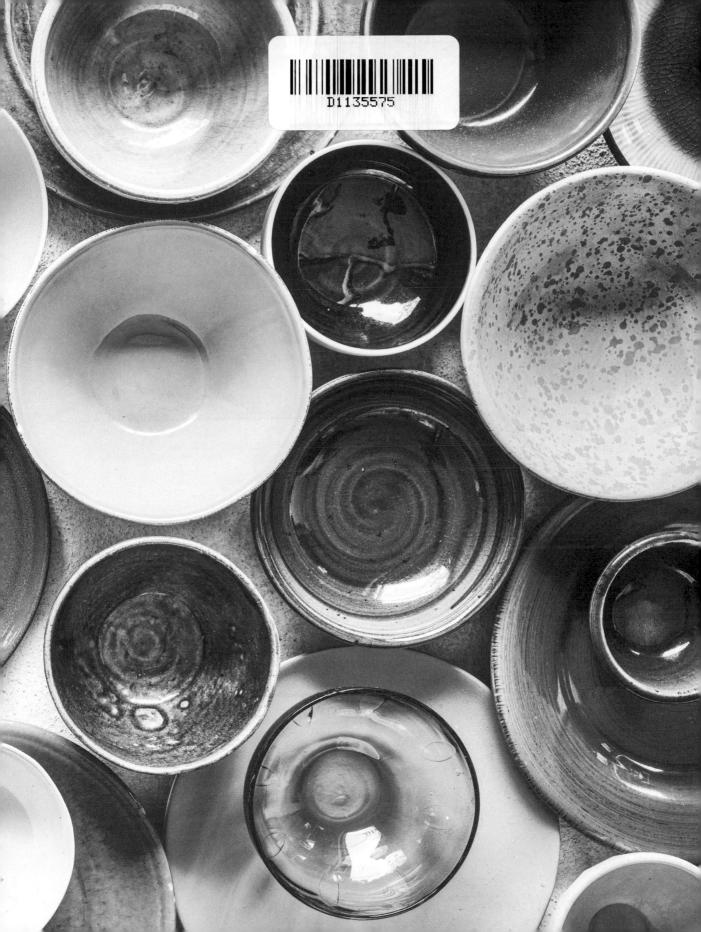

TWOCHUBBYCUBS

TWOCHUBBYCUBS
FAST AND FILLING

100 Delicious, Slimming Recipes

James Anderson & Paul Anderson

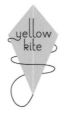

First published in Great Britain in 2020 by Yellow Kite
An imprint of Hodder & Stoughton
An Hachette UK company

2

Hardback ISBN 978 1 529 39809 0
eBook ISBN 978 1 529 39810 6

Colour origination by AltaImage
Printed in Germany by Firmengruppe APPL

Hodder & Stoughton policy is to use papers that are
natural, renewable and recyclable products and made
from wood grown in sustainable forests. The logging and
manufacturing processes are expected to conform to the
environmental regulations of the country of origin.

Yellow Kite
Hodder & Stoughton Ltd
Carmelite House
50 Victoria Embankment
London EC4Y 0DZ

www.yellowkitebooks.co.uk
www.hodder.co.uk

Notes

The information and references contained herein are
for informational purposes only. They are designed to
support, not replace, any ongoing medical advice given
by a healthcare professional and should not be construed
as the giving of medical advice nor relied upon as a basis
for any decision or action.

Readers should consult their doctor before altering their
diet, particularly if they are on a set diet prescribed by
their doctor or dietician.

The calorie count for each recipe is an estimate only
and may vary depending on the brand of ingredients
used, and due to the natural biological variations in
the composition of foods such as meat, fish, fruit and
vegetables. It does not include the nutritional content of
garnishes or any optional accompaniments recommended
for taste/serving in the ingredients list.

Where not specified, ingredients are analysed as average
or medium, not small or large. Eggs are medium, butter is
unsalted and milk is semi-skimmed unless otherwise stated.

Editoral Director: Lauren Whelan
Project Editor: Grace Paul
Copy-editor: Annie Lee
Proofreaders: Kay Halsey and Vicky Orchard
Nutritionist: Kerry Torrens
Internal Design: Clare Skeats
Photographers: Liz and Max Haarala Hamilton
Food Stylist: Frankie Unsworth
Prop Stylist: Charlie Phillips
Production Manager: Diana Talyanina
Deafening Spiritual Guidance: Dorothy Barron

CONTENTS

INTRODUCTION

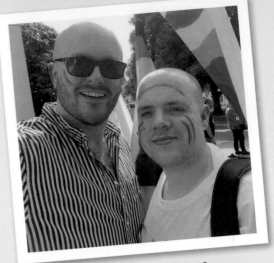

You'll see that neither of us can look at a camera

Oh hey! Fancy seeing you here!

Listen, I know I said I'd call you, but the thing is, life got in the way. The kids have been poorly and the other half has been sniffing around, you know how they get. It wasn't you, it was me, and that rash will go away if you just rub a little natural yoghurt on it. Only a little, mind, no one needs to see your hot-take on a Fruit Corner any time soon.

I jest, of course, I'd always call you back – just don't tell the others. We find ourselves back together at the dawn of a new book and may I say that you've never looked better?

We are the twochubbycubs, James and Paul, a married couple from Newcastle, and you'll know us via one of four ways:

★ You thoroughly enjoyed our last recipe book, plus our delightful diet planner, and have been waiting patiently for a sequel.

★ You have been following our blog for many years and still can't quite believe we managed to convince a publishing house to put our filth in print.

★ You bought this book because the cover was colourful and other books were out of stock.

★ You've been given this book by someone who liked you *just* enough to buy you a book but not enough to take you out for dinner.

A note before we get started. Although we are 'one', Paul is generally the poor sap who does the cooking and I, James, get to fanny about on the computer and bash out a few words every now and then. So, going forward, when the book refers to 'I', know that I am speaking for the both of us. Just like I do with Paul's test results or a second mortgage application on Chubby Towers.

The last year has been a whirlwind. To understand how we feel, know this about the two of us: we aren't chefs, and we've never run a restaurant or received classes or tuition from those that know how to cook. Indeed, the only time I've ever been lectured to by someone with a fancy white pinny was when I was being told off at the 'clinic' for being a promiscuous trollop.

We set up a blog many moons ago to post what we considered to be the antithesis to the slimming recipes that were being proffered up on social media: these recipes were always watery, miserable-looking affairs that dodged flavour and ingredients in the

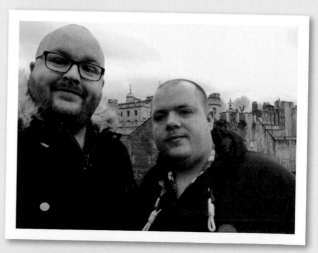

Us at our chunkiest, faking our smiles

name of being 'good for dieting'. We wanted food that was indulgent, easy to cook and, most important of all, didn't feel like 'diet food'. So, with all the earnestness that two fat lads can manage, we started creating the recipes ourselves, tinkering and tailoring as we went, to work out what tasted good. We posted the results online, people started following us, and we never looked back.

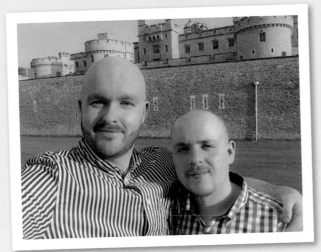

Us at our skinniest. Paul looks about thirteen

That's a fib, actually – we always look back, we don't want people stealing our silver.

We discovered our 'diet', such as it was, worked, and fuelled by a challenge on prime-time TV, we lost over eighteen stone. No gimmicks: just good food and a little bit of exercise. I asked if I could cheat and simply divorce Paul, losing seventeen stone in one fell swoop, but the producers demurred at my suggestion, saying it wouldn't make for good television. I disagree: we could have been the Geordie Den 'n' Angie – Paul would look damn good with a perm.

After the programme aired, we were approached by any number of publishers who asked us to do what our fans had been nagging us to do for years – write a book. We declined so many offers, until one very persistent Editorial Director made me laugh so much on a phone call that I immediately signed us up. We spent the next few months pulling together

our recipes, writing our nonsense and absolutely papping ourselves that the curtain would be pulled back and we would be revealed as the shams we thought we were.

If I can have a moment to take my hand off me ha'penny and pop it on my cholesterol-soaked heart: we didn't expect to sell. We thought a few people might buy the book out of politeness, pity or familial obligations, then straight into the shredder it would go. That's not false modesty, mind you, we just didn't think it would take off.

Boy, was my face red – and not just from the effort of signing all the autographed copies, mind you. It was a genuine, utter success, selling way past what we could have ever hoped for. It has been an incredible experience and one that we don't want to downplay here. It's a difficult feeling to put into words: when you've wanted to be an author all of your life, to see your own book in the shops is just beyond astounding. To have people take the time to write to you to say thank you, or to say they've never laughed so much at a cookbook, is lovely. Paul, for all his years of sweating in the kitchen (indeed, any situation at all), had people cooking his meals, showing off their dinners and just having fun again with their diet, and he was utterly delighted. I'm brash and can take a compliment, he's far more shy about realizing he's not that bad really.

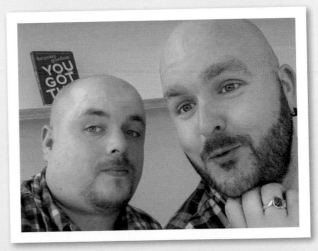

Our first publisher meeting: I'm wearing my horcrux

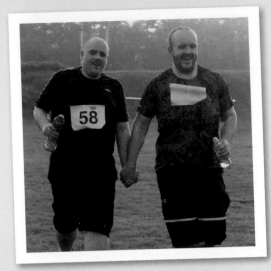

Running from the police after 'looking for badgers'

So, at this point, let us both say a giant, colossal and heartfelt thank you to everyone who has supported us, bought our book or said a kind word. You honestly have no idea how much you've changed our lives! Mind, Paul still hasn't got his conservatory or a dog, and I'm still as tight as a tick's nipsy, but we persevere.

Enough gushing, though. The book came out and we embarked on all sorts of thrilling escapades. Book signings were a particular highlight, although they got cut short when the pandemic swept the nation. A real shame … I was enjoying people swooning in my presence due to my chiselled (by a JCB) jaw and overly generous application of Tom Ford. The thought that people would get up early and queue up just to see our jolly faces was entirely alien to us – I wouldn't get out of bed early to throw a bucket of water on Paul if he was slightly on fire.

We signed books, we signed a pink dog, we even had a stab at signing a couple of boobs, though we had to draw a line when someone asked us to sign her apron pocket, which was positioned neatly over an area I'm not familiar enough with to confidently navigate. Plus, it was a good Sharpie and I didn't like to risk losing it. It turns out that we can find a myriad of different ways to say, 'What recipes are you looking

forward to?' and 'How far have you come?', and Paul's a surprisingly effortless raconteur – you think you know someone …

In the midst of all the excitement we learned that our book was to be featured on ITV's *Save Money: Lose Weight* programme, where some chubby wonder was to eat all our recipes all the time and see how much weight they lost. Now, we weren't told about this beforehand in the interest of keeping everything fair (Paul does rather have a look that suggests he could (a) sort you out some copper wiring or (b) get someone to put your kneecaps out) and so we were, to put it bluntly, papping ourselves when it aired.

Thankfully, there was no twist: our recipes were tested and, even better, the chap who was following our diet lost a tonne of weight. Better yet, the book came third of 'best overall diets' and even then was only pushed into third by two 'fad' diets. Mind, one of those involved swallowing a teaspoon or so of suspiciously viscous slightly off-white liquid every day: well, I've been doing that (and then some!) for over two decades now and I'm still very much a chubby cub. It's the lies I can't handle.

We had no time to celebrate the victory, however, for we were due to go and record a segment on *James Martin's Saturday Morning* the very next day. Let me explain: James Martin is a personal hero of the both of us – the way that man commands a knob of butter is heaven to us. Plus, no discretion here, he's an absolute stunner. We care not for being subtle here at twochubbycubs.

We were originally due to record with Beverley Callard (that's Liz from *Coronation Street*, mind) and were utterly cock-a-hoop to not only meet James but Liz too, but sadly she got swapped for Matthew Kelly. That isn't to say he was anything short of delightful because I'm sure he was, but when I think of what might have been …

Saturday came round then, as it is wont to do, and there's us rolling up at James's own house, full of nerves and skyrocketing impostor syndrome. We always say we aren't proper chefs – look at the start of this intro – and yet here we were being asked to prepare a dish on TV with a man who is a legend in the world of cuisine. Thankfully, they took the pressure off us a little by asking us to 'assemble' a dish rather than having to cook anything, while James talked to us about the cookbook.

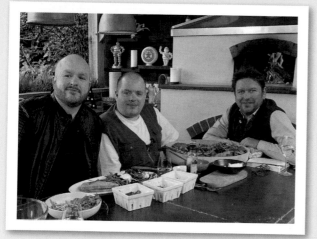

I was too cool for a waistcoat

We were rushed through make-up. I was only in for a minute, and most of that was the make-up artist crying and saying she could never touch such perfection, whereas Paul was in for two hours and they had to helicopter a team over from *Embarrassing Bodies* (I jest, it was *Ground Force*), and then we were straight into recording.

We had elected to make the Berry Berry Salad dish from the last book because it's a doddle to put a salad together, surely? It's simply a matter of plating up the different elements, pouring over the sauce and presenting it with a camp flourish. What could go wrong? To assist us, the Home Economist backstage (a lovely lady from round our way) chopped and presented all the constituent parts. As I'm Chief Gasbag and thus would be altogether too busy making moony-eyes at James and answering all his questions with flirty laughter, Paul was asked to prepare the salad.

Cameras rolling, and off we go. Five minutes passed of us answering questions, giggling and me trying to work out which bedroom in James' house I'd be using as my walk-in wardrobe, when James suggested Paul start making the salad. Paul did, getting the mixing bowl and tipping every last leaf he had in front of him into it. There was probably enough greenery there to feed sixteen people, pushed into a bowl made for four. I could see his panic out of the corner of my eye but tried to smooth it out by laughing gaily and talking louder, in much the same way I get through funerals of loved ones.

Paul, a man whose entire life mantra is 'push on regardless', was trying to get his porky hands into the bowl to toss this salad, but couldn't. I knew there was trouble when the tip of his tongue appeared in the corner of his mouth – a sure sign that his brain is working at full capacity and about to overheat. Clearly realizing he had boobed, he decided to go all in and chucked all the berries on top of this towering pile of leaves. At this point I could see James's polite smile betray just a hint of 'what the hell is he doing' and he stepped in, pulling a giant paella pan from behind him and offering it up as a rescue.

Paul gratefully accepted and to his credit managed to make a perfectly good-looking salad in the end, albeit one that could feed the entire country of Uzbekistan and still have some left over. We would go down on record as the two fat lads with a *Sunday Times*-bestselling cookbook who couldn't make a bloody salad.

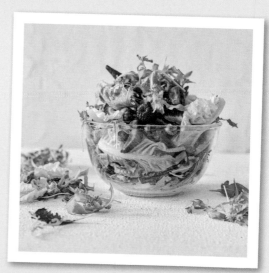

Paul's second attempt at making the salad

9

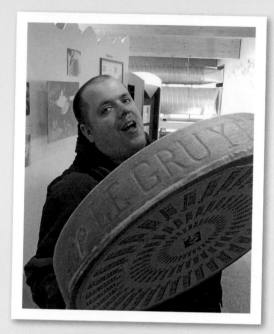

When two become one

The timing point is particularly important this time because for this book we have focused on three main themes:

★ Food that doesn't taste like diet food but just so happens to be healthy.

★ Food that doesn't take an age to prepare or cook.

★ Or if it does take a while to cook, it'll be bloody easy to batch cook and portion up the leftovers.

We know you don't always have time to cook lavish meals and spend hours stirring away in the kitchen. Plus, it's not always about time – sometimes you just can't be arsed. We hear you, and that's why all the recipes in here are designed to make your life a little easier. We've included symbols to show fast recipes, recipes that are easy to scale up, recipes that freeze well. We've also upped the vegetarian recipes ever so slightly, but every single meal in here is one to enjoy wherever you stand.

Readers, the internet comments were bloody awful. But see, if we cared about what people who kvetch on the internet thought of us, we'd never get anything done. As it happens, Paul – awash with humility – apologized to James off-air and mentioned that we had no right being there. In what was a moment that made even my granite heart sing, he was told he had as much right to be there as any chef, and we got to scribble our names on the wall of guests. You know who would have been proud? Liz.

And that was that. Unfortunately, not long after, the country went into lockdown and everything stopped – bar one thing. Pleas for a sequel. Well, never let it be said that we can't satisfy you twice over, despite our advancing years, because here it is!

In preparation for the sequel we have done a little market research to find out what you lot want. Let us lead with a couple of new additions to this book. We have remembered to include exactly how long the recipes take to cook this time, after totally forgetting this in the last book. We've also included a piece on 'storecupboard staples' because we know it helps folks to be able to take stock of what they have.

But most importantly, we've tried to give you more of what you loved from the last book, and what you enjoy about the blog. These are meals that we eat with stories about us. We appreciate that some folks like to sit and read a recipe book for the food stories, but honestly, there's so many of those out there that we have tried to stay different.

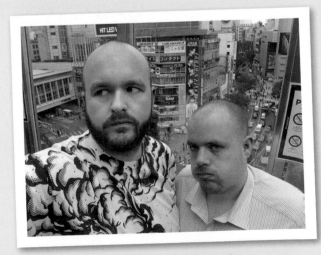

We always thoroughly enjoy ourselves wherever we go

So, this, then, is our book. Our second chapter. The difficult second album, only we aren't experimenting with awful new routes: just more of the same. We wanted to call the book 'twochubbycubs come again', but the publisher said nay. Fair do's: fast and filling does rather suit us.

We hope you enjoy every word and savour every meal you cook. There's nothing in here that will give you difficulty in terms of cooking, but even if it does, don't fret: cooking should be fun, not some awful exercise in stress and panic. If your end results don't look like ours, who cares? Eat it, I bet it still tastes lovely. Good luck with your cooking and dieting and please do get in touch with us to let us know what you think. We're on all the usual social media streams: see our handles below. We always try to respond personally because you know, we bloody love hearing from you and frankly, if you've deigned to open your purse and slip us some money, it's the least we can do.

Without further delay, then.

With love and endless pride,

JAMES & PAUL

PS: The mystery of the half-potato from the last book? Where I explained that when I went to my nana's she would have half a potato in a jug of water on the side, and she rudely died before we ever got a satisfactory explanation as to what she was doing?

You came through for us with a myriad of different reasons: perhaps she was making 'starchy' water for ironing with? Definitely not: her clothes were as wrinkly as the skin around her sparkling eyes when she smiled, which was so very often. Others suggested she was softening up the potato to make better chips, but that, I'm afraid, is a nonsense too. She may have had a full set of NHS dentures, but she never needed anything mushing up.

No, I'm afraid the answer is far simpler: it was an air-freshener, way back from a time when plug-ins and deodorizers weren't a thing. She's up in the clouds somewhere now so I can get away with this, but Nana, love, it didn't work. We knew when your famous poached cod (steady on, she was in her eighties) was ready by the sheer overpowering waft hitting us – and we lived two miles away. Bless her. We miss her magnificently.

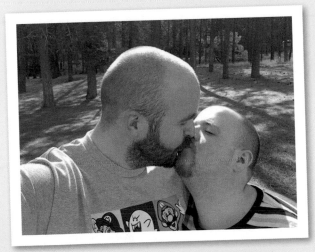

This isn't romance, Paul just had a bit of pancake in his teeth that I fancied

KEEP IN TOUCH AND TAG US WITH YOUR TASTY CREATIONS!

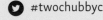 twochubbycubs 　 @twochubbycubs 　 #twochubbycubs

HOW TO USE THE BOOK

The new key, exciting aspect of this book – following our market research and answering the endless questions and comments from the last book – is that we have included a handy set of symbols to assist you when making a decision on what recipe to cook. Naturally, because all of our recipes are simple and delicious, you'll want to cook all the recipes anyway, but we're nothing if not all about making your life easier.

The symbols are all new bar the star symbol, which carries over from the last book – recipes that are starred are recipes that featured on the blog to critical acclaim. I say critical, it was mainly my mother ringing up, slurring her words and asking us to cook it for her because she'd had one too many Camparis. Ah, life. Mind, we had to make sure we answered the 'star' question because we entirely neglected to explain it in the previous book, leading to some overly enthusiastic readers thinking we'd included some kind of exciting mystery to solve. Alas no: we were just at deadline and were too busy spending the royalties. Our mistake. But you love us for it.

The overall theme to our recipes this year is that they are fast, filling or a delightful combination of the two. Now, that doesn't automatically mean they are fast to cook – sometimes they may take a little longer to prepare but are easy to batch cook or freeze well afterwards. So time spent now means time saved later, and isn't that just a wonder?

You will see from our recipes that we believe in spending 'calories' on proper ingredients and we very rarely use 'low fat' or 'fat free' unless the recipe works well with them. Please, don't be too aghast by some of the suggestions: if these meals are your main meal of the day, then it is absolutely worth spending the calories. That said: they're all under 500 calories! Under the calories on each recipe you'll also find 'diet' which indicates if something is vegetarian (VEG), vegan (V), gluten-free (GF) or dairy-free (DF), because we're thoughtful like that.

OH! One final note. All calorie amounts for the recipes are per person, not per meal. I know, it's a disappointment, but we did have one reader chastise us for the last book because they had been eating for six. Everything in moderation …

BLOG Some of our most-loved blog recipes that we go back to time and time again.

EASY TO SCALE UP These are your go-to recipes when you have an hour or so and you want to prepare enough for as many servings as you like – the recipes lend themselves to doubling or tripling the ingredients without any major dramas.

QUICK TO MAKE The prep and cooking takes 30 minutes combined or less for these recipes – perfect when you can't be chewed on standing in front of the oven.

GOOD FOR LUNCHES Lunches are an absolute knacker when you're on a diet, so we've tried to include some recipes that are just the ticket for taking into the office or, in these uncertain times, taking into the next room of your house and pretending you're in the office – it's that easy.

FREEZES WELL I mean, come on, that one doesn't need explaining!

ONE PAN Be it in a frying pan or a roasting tin, easy one-pan meals that'll save time afterwards when you're not washing the carving knife and wondering whether or not you'd do well in prison – just me?

DIETARY We want to ensure that we cater for everyone's needs and are aware that lots of people have different diets, so we've flagged which recipes are vegetarian (VEG), vegan (V), gluten-free (GF) and dairy-free (DF) for readers. Because we care.

STORECUPBOARD STAPLES

A well-stocked cupboard, aside from a forgiving husband and a fire blanket, is probably the most important thing you need when you're cooking: and this applies doubly if you're shifting a bit of gut at the same time, because goodness knows we need to replace all that nice-tasting fat with other flavours. Please don't look at this list and immediately clutch your pearls – there's no need to go out and buy them all at once: pick up maybe one or two each time you go shopping and you'll be fine. Looking through the list, you can probably pick out a few that you know you'll use often – start with those. Once you start building up what you have, your food horizons will expand significantly. Eeh, listen to us, honestly, we forget that we both came from houses with pay-as-you-go tellies.

But it's true. One of the best things we ever bought when we started the blog was a spice rack, bursting with flavours and ideas. We then got rid of the spice rack in favour of some fancy magnetic jars on the side of the fridge, which work an absolute treat until you come in from a night out absolutely steaming, fall against your fridge and end up on the floor covered in turmeric. Paul thought I was doing some weird Simpsons role-play, I was just trying not to vomit up 20g of paprika.

One tip with your spices: keep them dry and dark, and rotate them out on a semi-regular basis. Spices lose their flavour and never more so than when they're sitting in sunlight for seventy months. Use your nose (are they pungent?) and your eyes (have the colours dulled?) and, if all else fails, simply hurl them at your partner to gauge their reaction.

One more tip, actually: you needn't go for the fancy, branded stuff – ours are all cobbled together with supermarket own brands and other knock-offs. It doesn't have to cost you a lot of money. World food sections and local shops are your best friends here.

That's the spices covered, but of course, a touch of spice is very nice but there's a myriad of other go-to ingredients we use a lot of. With that in mind, Paul has split our favourites into several groups, which he thinks you'll find helpful. He's also given them ridiculous group names because he's a touch 'live, laugh, love' at the moment, much to my chagrin. It's funny how someone so beautiful can be so wrong, isn't it? Remember, we're not precious about our cooking: if you're doing a recipe and find you haven't got an ingredient that you need, try swapping it with something similar in that group. Do it your way. The key to good cooking is to be unafraid of throwing caution to the

14

wind and mixing up the recipe – as long as you're replacing 'like for like', you really shouldn't go too wrong.

Of course, now we've said that, there's gonna be a plethora of people foaming at the mouth because they replaced the pesto in our pesto burgers with Castrol GTX, aren't there? Sigh. A writer's work is never silent. Let's get to it.

SPICES

The Warmers and the Tinglers

Paprika/smoked paprika/sweet
     paprika (if you're getting just
     one, go for the smoked paprika)
Cayenne pepper
Hot chilli powder
Dried chilli flakes

The Curry Ones

Ground cumin
Ground turmeric
Garam masala
Mild/hot curry powder

The (Pumpkin) Spice Gals

Five spice
Ground nutmeg
Ground cinnamon
Ground allspice
Ground ginger
Fennel seeds

The 'Pack a Punch' Ones

Cajun
Jerk

HERBS

The Nice Aromatic Ones

Dried mixed herbs
Dried oregano
Dried thyme
Dried dill
Dried rosemary
Dried parsley

The Deep Crooners

Ground coriander
Dried sage
Dried tarragon
Dried rosemary
Bay leaves

OTHERS

The Backing Singers

Onion powder/granules
Garlic powder/granules
Cracked black pepper
Salt

PASTA & GRAINS

When it comes to pastas and grains, you'll be well versed already. In any of our pasta recipes, feel free to swap them out with whatever you have in your cupboard. Grains and rices can be swapped too, but just be sure to check the cooking times – they can sometimes vary. These will last an age in your cupboards. We like to decant them into glass Kilner jars – it makes it easier to see what we have and creates a nice focal point by the bin when we realize we've stockpiled eighteen years' worth of risotto rice by accident.

OILS

We use olive oil in our recipes unless specified otherwise. It's a good all-rounder. Sunflower, groundnut (peanut) and vegetable oils are fine alternatives. Sesame oil is great to have in the cupboard too but used more in our recipes to add flavour. Flavoured oils have their place, but make sure you buy decent varieties – we recommend Yorkshire Drizzle (we aren't paid to say that, mind, they're just bloody good), but you can shop around.

SAUCES, PASTES & VINEGARS

We're betting you'll have most of these in your cupboard already, but if not, do grab whatever you need next time you're out. Most of them will last ages if stored properly, and are perfect for slopping in your meals for a bit of bang. It goes without saying that ketchup, brown sauce and all the usual condiments should be stocked up in the cupboard.

A note on fish sauce especially: it smells absolutely revolting. Like someone has already had a crack at digesting it and set it aside for a poorly cat. But it makes certain dishes sing: try your best to get over your gag reflex. Ring James if you need assistance on that front.

Sriracha
Oyster sauce
Hoisin sauce
Soy sauce (light/dark/
    reduced-sodium/normal)
Worcestershire sauce
Dijon mustard

Chilli bean paste
Balsamic vinegar
Fish sauce
Cider vinegar
Rice vinegar
Rice wine vinegar
Mirin

TOMATOES & TINS

When it comes to tomatoes, we use good passata and flavour it ourselves, but there's no shame in buying the flavoured varieties. Make sure you taste your tomato dishes as you go – a touch of sugar can change the meal completely. Always keep a good stock of tinned tomatoes (plum and chopped) to hand.

Similarly, pulses from a tin are nothing to be ashamed of. Adding a tin of pulses to a meal can stretch it further, and they're perfect for chucking into a slow-cooker stew.

OTHER BITS & BOBS

Stock cubes are one of the rare things we encourage getting a 'higher brand' of – good stock can make a meal, so don't be tight. If you can make your own, even better!

Panko breadcrumbs
Baking powder
Cornflour
Plain flour/self-raising flour
Walnuts/chopped dry-roasted
    peanuts/hazelnuts

Granulated sugar/
    brown sugar
Honey
Maple syrup
Vanilla extract
Porridge oats

Panko are a type of breadcrumb with a larger surface area and 'lighter' than usual. They make things crunchier and they're bloody lovely and I swear if anyone else asks me what bloody panko is, I'll do time. You can find them in most large supermarkets – if you're struggling, just use normal breadcrumbs.

FABULOUS FREEZING

....

We get asked ever so much about which gadgets bring us joy, and while my answer involves a sculpted piece of rubber about the size of a caravan fire-extinguisher and which plugs straight into the National Grid, Paul will answer with a freezer. Hear him out.

Almost all of us have a freezer, and yet how do we use it? We cram it full of nonsense from the supermarkets and only ever take stock of what we have in there when the act of finding space for one garden pea becomes a protracted three-hour affair. How many bags of mixed vegetables do you have in there right now that haven't seen the light of day since 2011? If you say less than four, then you're a shameful liar.

You know just by looking at us that we aren't ones for leftovers generally – we had to buy plastic plates because Paul was taking the shine off the 'proper' plates from scraping every last morsel of food off there. But, when you're dieting and being economical with food, a freezer is a wonderful thing when used right.

So, in the spirit of giving, we have provided some top tips to help you make the most of your freezer and to turn it into a wonderful igloo of delicious meals and tasty memories, but we also give a note of caution: if you're unsure of anything you are freezing or defrosting, take the time to double check online what you're supposed to be doing. Spending four hours on the lavatory sobbing into a toilet roll may be great for weight loss, but it is also exceptionally dangerous. You be careful, I dare say we've grown fond of you.

FEEL THE HEAT

Moist foods like stews and casseroles cook well from frozen. We start them off at a lower temperature and then turn the dial up to complete the cook. Covering the food with a sheet of foil or an ovenproof lid will stop the surface of the food from browning too much. Other dishes that work well from frozen are soups and potato-topped pies. Never cook raw poultry or large joints of meat from frozen, always defrost in the fridge first.

NICE RICE BABY

At Chubby Towers we usually make enough rice for a rugby team when cooking for tea. We are forever optimistic. You can freeze the excess but you have to be bloody careful. Cool the rice quickly, ideally within an hour (tip it into a shallow container to cool down), and then freeze. To re-use, defrost the rice in the fridge, cook through until steaming hot – but do this just the once. If you're re-heating in the microwave, add a few tablespoons of water.

DADDY, CHILL

Don't be throwing hot food into your cold freezer. The temperature of the freezer will rise and you might ruin all your previous efforts. Plus, you might burn out the freezer motor, and then won't you feel a silly billy?

PUT SOMETHING ON THE END OF IT

Store your food in freezer-friendly, sealed containers or airtight bags. This should stop freezer burn – that's the frosty layer which forms over the surface of the food when it's in contact with air or Paul's bad attitude. Freezer burn causes the food to discolour and just isn't pleasant. Use square or rectangular containers to make sure there's no wasted space. Plus: don't forget water expands when it freezes, so any liquids or saucy dishes need about 1cm headspace to allow for this.

A TOUCH OF DEFROST

Always defrost foods thoroughly and use within 24 hours, like you're a Poundland Jack Bauer. Defrost in a cool place like the fridge, pantry or the fashion scene of Amsterdam. Defrosting raw fish or meat? Stand it on a bowl or plate to catch any thawed liquid, and keep it away from other food, or so help me God. Then, when it's time to cook, cook it until it's steaming hot and only reheat once.

DIVIDE & STONKER

It's so much easier to divide your leftovers into the correct portion sizes before freezing, unless you're a dab hand with the chainsaw. Wouldn't surprise us, mind.

GUESS WHO?

Label your leftovers, including whether it's cooked or has gone in raw. This eliminates the game of desfrosting something to see what it is and realizing you've got half a tiramisu to serve with your dirty rice.

TIME WAITS FOR NO HAM

Freezing food is like pressing the pause button but most experts suggest 3–6 months as the rule of thumb for keeping your frozen food. After this time, food tends to lose flavour and it'll be safe, but if it isn't like a taste explosion in your mouth, what's the point in eating it? So make sure to add the date to the label.

ON THE FLOP

Some foods don't like the cold and will turn limp, slushy or rubbery without a thought for your feelings. Avoid hard-boiled eggs, egg yolks, mayo and egg-containing sauces as well as high water veggies like lettuce, tomatoes, cucumber or beansprouts. It's also best to steer clear of stuffed poultry, from a food safety point of view.

REFREEZER? WE BARELY KNEW 'ER!

Freezing food is a great way to preserve leftovers as well to avoid food waste. However, there are some rules you'll need to follow and your mantra should always be 'if in doubt don't'. Generally speaking it's fine to cook frozen raw meat and fish and then refreeze the cooked dish but don't refreeze meat or fish which is raw or cooked food that has already been frozen and defrosted.

OUR KITCHEN TIPS

Years of watching Paul sweat away in the kitchen has afforded me the luxury of being able to tut furiously, lean in and 'give advice' and tell him exactly what he is doing wrong. It's a fantastic feeling and one that I have been able to take advantage of many times over, much to his eternal chagrin. With that in mind, and with some input (mostly swearing and telling me he's the cook and I'm the writer and I ought to know my place) from Paul, on the opposite page there are a few snippets of IMPORTANT THINGS to remember when you're cooking.

We were asked to put a photo of us laughing and joking in the kitchen here, but given we spend most of our time in the kitchen hurling pans at each other and screaming, we thought it would be better to include a picture of our cats.

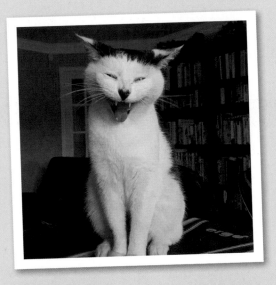

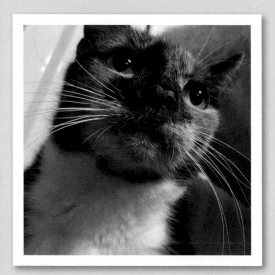

This is Bowser. Bowser likes eating bees and then coming in with a swollen face like he's been out fighting lorries. This was the best picture we had of him, and it works.

This is Sola, and you must understand that she has absolutely no time for your kitchen calamities. You either do what she says without question or you'll find yourself buried up to your eyes in the cat litter box.

A DROPPED KNIFE HAS NO HANDLE

I can't begin to tell you the amount of times I've seen Paul drop a knife and rush to catch it, only for it to go spectacularly wrong. It's why sometimes I look down during Fun Time and think Freddy Krueger is having a pull on me. If you drop a knife – indeed, anything – let it hit the floor. You can always pick it up, which you can't do if your fingers have been severed and rolled behind the cat litter box.

LEARN HOW HOT YOUR OVEN RUNS

If there's one thing I've learned as a flamboyant gay man it's that just because you've turned the knob correctly, doesn't mean the end result is great. Some ovens run a little hotter than others, so buy yourself an ovenproof thermometer and check that the temperature you're cooking at is what you imagined.

DON'T BLOODY RUSH

Paul's an absolute knacker for doing this, he really is. If a recipe calls for gently frying the onions for example, don't go boiling them away for a couple of minutes just so you can have a sit-down – all the best things take time.

DON'T OVERCROWD IT

If you're frying or sautéing in a pan, jam that pan to the brim and you'll simply be steaming your food, which just won't work. I know we're all here reading this book because we're not overly patient and cautious when it comes to food, but taking things slowly and cooking food in batches is no bad thing, I swear.

LEAVE THE LID ON

If you're cooking rice in a pan (i.e. it's not microwave rice, you slattern) then for goodness sake, leave the lid on while it cooks. Rice cooks in the steam, and by lifting the lid off to 'check on it', you're ruining everything and ought to be thoroughly ashamed.

BUY CHEAP, BUY TWICE

While there truly isn't a need to spend a lot of money on kitchen gadgets and gizmos, if you are buying a new pan or knife set, do your research and buy the best you can afford. Replacing a £2.99 knife made of mist and dreams eight times over is a false economy.

BUY THE BEST MAIN INGREDIENT

We stress this throughout the book, but if a recipe is simple, then make sure you buy the best of the main ingredient that you can. We always turn to tomatoes for this – vine-ripened tomatoes left in the sun, none of your 'at least it's red' jobs from the supermarket.

YOU CAN ALWAYS ADD MORE BUT YOU CAN'T TAKE AWAY

This applies to many things (insults, scars across your marriage vows, etc.) but none more so than seasoning. When you're cooking, add a little and then taste – if you go pouring salt on your food like you're trying to hold back an oil slick, you can easily ruin the whole dish. If you do it in little pinches here and there, well, you'll be cooking on gas. Or electric. Maybe induction if you're fancy.

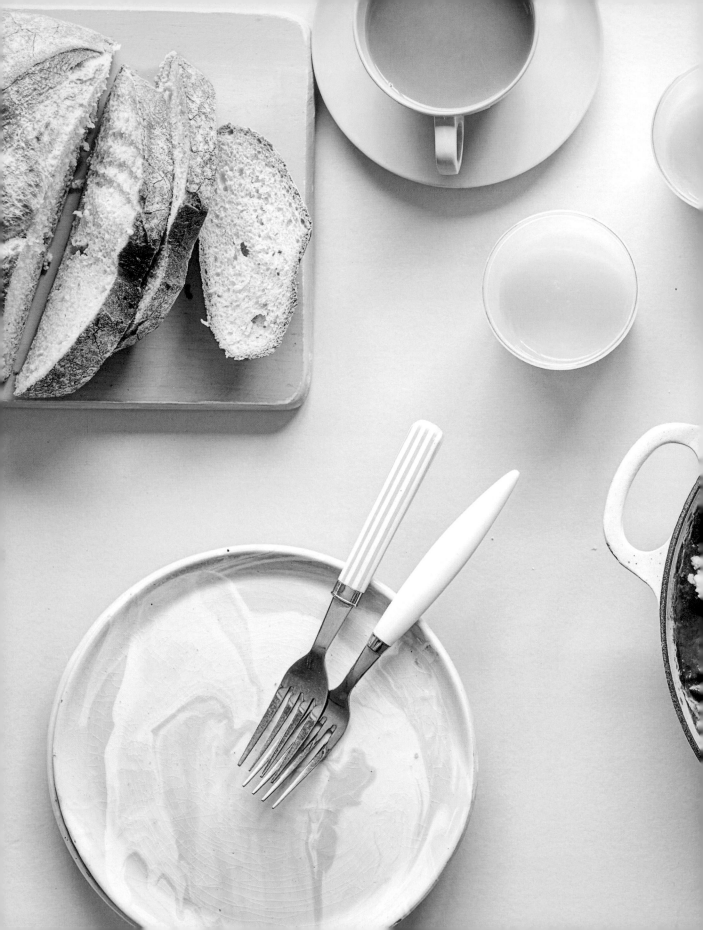

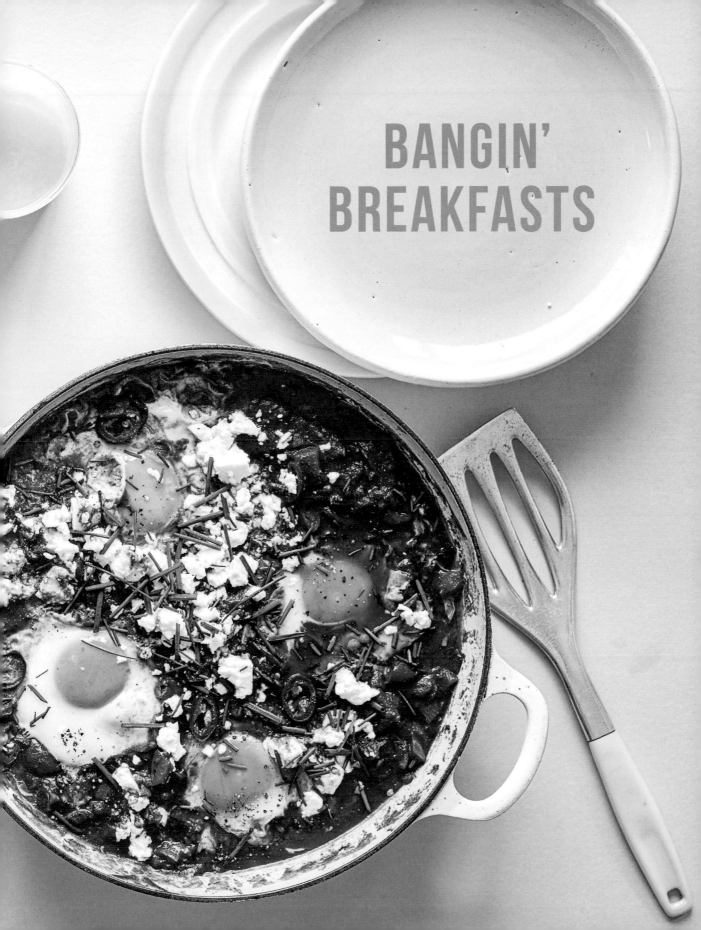

BANGIN' BREAKFASTS

BLUEBERRY PIE PORRIDGE

SERVES: 4
PREP: 5 minutes
COOK: 15 minutes
CALORIES: 335
DIET: VEG

There's a lot to be said for a steaming bowl of porridge to set you up for the day. Although we recommend blueberries, you can swap them for raspberries or strawberries – we tend to keep mixed berries in the freezer for just this occasion.

Mornings are always a fraught affair in our house: Paul likes to lie in bed until the sun goes back down at any opportunity, whereas I am very much an early bird. Years of looking after our cats, Bowser and Sola, have created this monster. See, at around 5 a.m. the cats decide they've really had quite enough of seeing us comfortably ensconced in bed and immediately set about clawing at my head, purring in my ear and, more disconcertingly, positioning themselves so the first thing I see when I wake up is their puckering bumholes a few inches from my eyes.

They're unbearably fussy, too: they'll go weeks snaffling away whatever we put in front of them only to abruptly decide that the food we offer them simply won't do. Given they spend most of their time licking their nethers, they're surprisingly snooty. If only I could communicate 'we saved you from a skip, show some gratitude' in cat language, it might knock them down a peg or two. But we do love them ever so much – as much as you'll love this porridge.

200g (7oz) frozen blueberries
500ml (18fl oz) unsweetened
   almond milk
180g (6½oz) porridge oats
1 banana
2 tbsp honey
½ tsp ground cinnamon
2 tbsp raisins
120g (4¼oz) natural yoghurt

Put the blueberries into a small saucepan and place over a medium heat. Stir frequently and simmer for about 10 minutes.

Meanwhile, put 500ml (18fl oz) of water into a large pan with the almond milk and bring to the boil.

Add the porridge oats and reduce the heat to low.

Mash the banana and add to the porridge pan, along with the honey, cinnamon and raisins.

Stir well, then simmer for another 6–8 minutes until the porridge reaches the consistency you like.

Spoon the porridge into bowls and top with the yoghurt and warm blueberries.

NOTE

This is perfectly scalable – for one person just quarter everything.

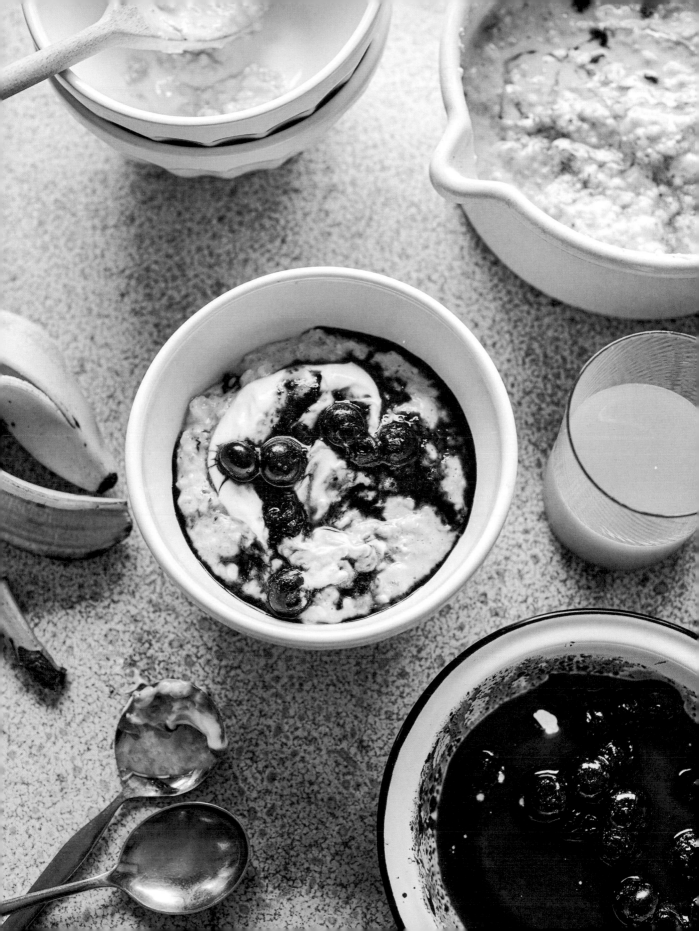

5 OVERNIGHT OATS RECIPES

Breakfast is always a struggle when you're after something fast and filling, but overnight oats should be your go-to meal when you're cutting a dash of a morning. Below we suggest five of our favourites, but don't you stop there – reach for the stars!

Oh, and I'd say this doesn't need to be said but, following feedback from our last book, perhaps it actually does: mix your oats together the night before. They'll not soften unless they're wet, rather like a good proportion of our readers …

SERVES: 1
PREP: 2 minutes
COOK: 0 minutes
CALORIES: 270
DIET: VEG

HOW TO MAKE THE BASE OATS MIXTURE

40g (1½oz) porridge oats
200g (7oz) fat-free natural yoghurt

Mix together and use as a base for any of the recipes below.

SERVES: 1
PREP: 5 minutes
COOK: 10 seconds
CALORIES: 384
DIET: VEG

STRAWBERRIES & CREAM

5 strawberries (plus 1 for the top)
a good few squirts of squirty cream

Chop the strawberries and muddle half of them with half of the base oats mixture.

Microwave the remaining strawberries for 10 seconds, then mash lightly with a fork.

Spoon the oats from the first step into a glass or bowl, and top with the microwaved strawberries and the rest of the oats.

Finish with the squirty cream and the extra strawberry.

SERVES: 1
PREP: 5 minutes
COOK: 0 minutes
CALORIES: 405
DIET: VEG

JAFFA CAKE

1 chocolate mini roll
3 tbsp mandarin segments in juice,
    drained

Chop the mini roll roughly and set aside.

Mix the base oats mixture with the mandarin segments and spoon into a glass or bowl.

Top with the chopped mini roll.

SERVES: 1
PREP: 5 minutes
COOK: 0 minutes
CALORIES: 288
DIET: VEG

(PAM) ST CLEMENTS

3 tbsp mandarin segments in juice,
    drained
zest and juice of ½ lemon (plus 1 slice
    for the top)

Mix the mandarin segments, lemon zest and juice with the base oats mixture and spoon into a glass or bowl.

Top with a slice of lemon for fanciness.

SERVES: 1
PREP: 5 minutes
COOK: 0 minutes
CALORIES: 493
DIET: VEG

MINT CHOC CHIP

40g (1½oz) milk chocolate chips
2 tsp peppermint extract
1 tsp green food colouring (optional)

Mix everything together with the base oats mixture.

Spoon into a glass or bowl.

SERVES: 1
PREP: 5 minutes
COOK: 0 minutes
CALORIES: 286
DIET: VEG

FRUITS OF THE FOREST

2 strawberries, chopped
1 tbsp raspberries
1 tbsp blackberries
1 tbsp blueberries

Muddle the fruit together and mix half with the base oats mixture.

Spoon into a glass or bowl and top with the remaining fruit.

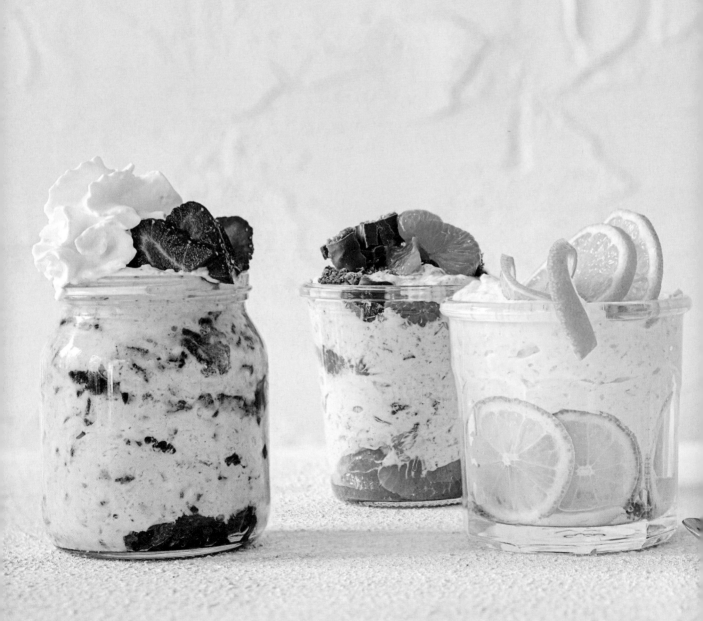

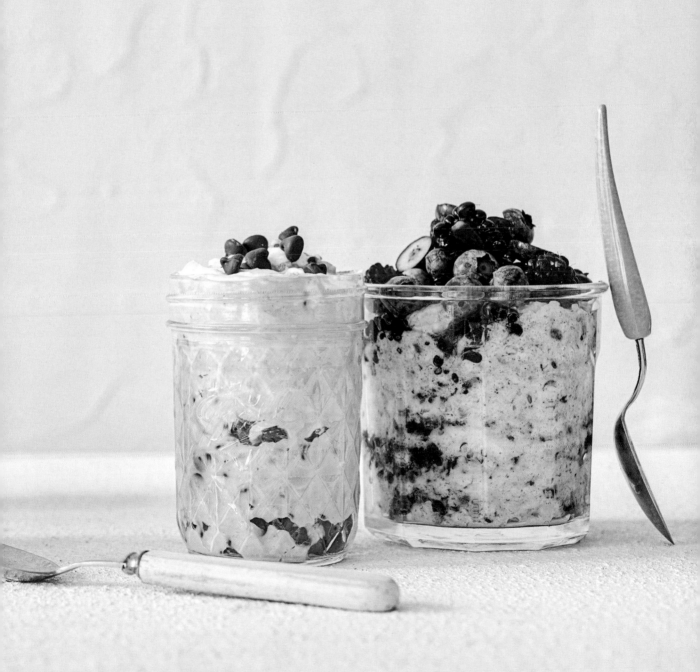

CHUBBY FRENCH TOAST

SERVES: 4
PREP: 10 minutes
COOK: 16 minutes
CALORIES: 340
DIET: VEG

At the time of writing this book, Paul and I are holed up in a fabulous Quayside hotel while Chubby Towers is getting a facelift. That makes everything sound terribly glamorous, but I remind you it's Newcastle in the fog, we're not talking summer in Tuscany. Which, in all honesty, is a frightful shame: I could do with a few months of finding myself and rolling around in fragrant hay with a baker called Alessandro who feared my love but embraced it none the less.

I digress. The reason I mention this is because one of the perks of being back in the city is the ability to use takeaway delivery services again: Chubby Towers is many things (notorious, crusted over, condemned), but it isn't well-connected. We have two takeaways available to us, and one of them we no longer use because we drove past once and saw the chef scratching his arse with such vim and vigour that we can only assume he'd lost something critical in there.

But, praise be: we can get breakfast delivered here, and we've been living on French toast like the two decadent bitches that we always knew we'd become. Here we present a slimming-friendly version, and we encourage you to make it a regular part of your life.

4 eggs
450ml (16fl oz) milk
¼ tsp ground cinnamon
8 slices of wholemeal bread
16 strawberries, cut into quarters
4 tsp honey
4 tbsp fat-free Greek yoghurt

Beat the eggs and milk together and add the cinnamon.

Dip each slice of bread into the egg mix and leave for a few seconds to soak in, then remove and lay on a plate.

Spray a large frying pan with a little oil and place it over a high heat.

Add the slices of bread to the pan in batches and cook for 1 minute, then turn and cook for another minute. Turn again and cook for 1 more minute, then turn and cook for a final minute – 4 minutes total.

Serve on a plate and top with the strawberries, honey and a tablespoon of yoghurt.

NOTE

For the best results, cook 2 slices at a time.

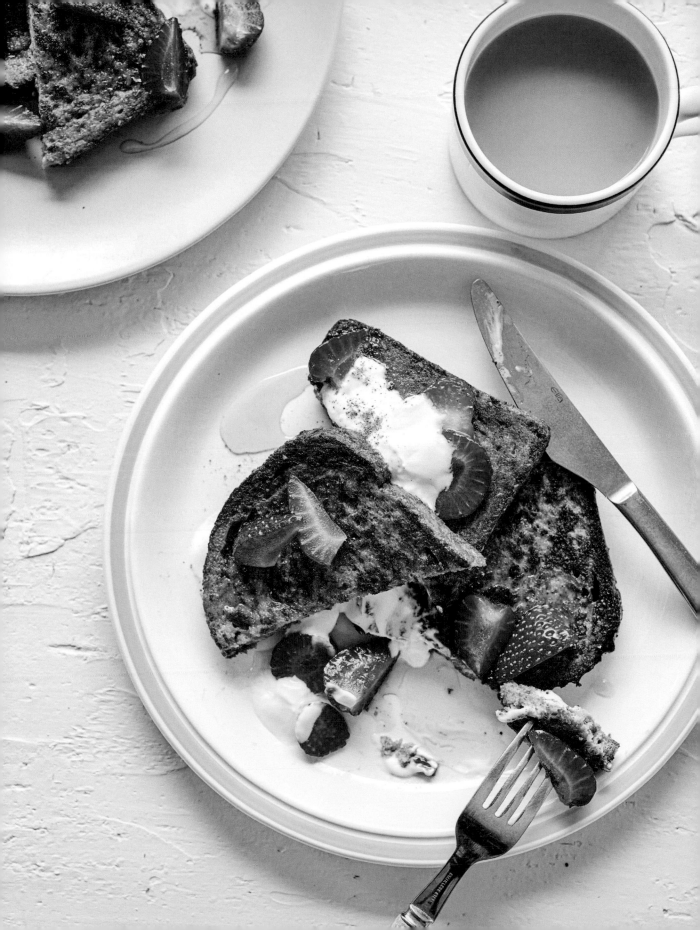

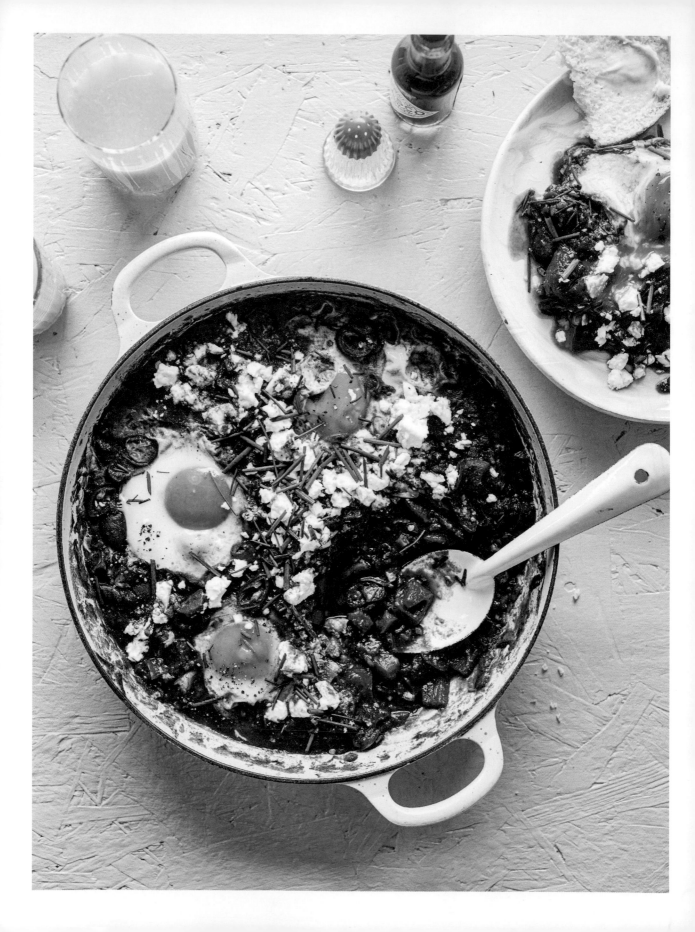

SHAKSHOUKA

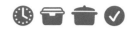

SERVES: 4
PREP: 5 minutes
COOK: 20 minutes
CALORIES: 200
DIET: VEG/GF

1 onion, finely diced
1 red pepper, sliced
1 small red chilli, finely diced
4 cloves of garlic, crushed
1 tsp ground cumin
1 tsp paprika
a pinch of salt
2 × 400g (14oz) tins of peeled
    plum tomatoes
4 large eggs
75g (2¾oz) feta cheese, crumbled
a handful of fresh chives,
    chopped

Did you know that shakshouka is the noise I make when I sneeze into Paul's beard when he's been too lax and carefree with the black pepper? Of course you didn't, unless you've been stalking us.

Mind, that's a sensitive subject: we actually did have a stalker of sorts for a good few months. It was entirely accidental, I'm sure, but it felt like whenever we went grocery shopping, there she was. She would bounce over, tut at everything in our trolley, jab me in the sides and say how fat I was getting, before disappearing into not exactly thin air. We called her Mrs Thrush and I'll let you decide why that was. Thankfully, she's dead now – that's right, dead tired of shopping at Waitrose so she's gone to pastures cheaper.

We've sidetracked. Shakshouka is an entirely forgiving breakfast that you can chuck all sorts into – I like to add cubed sweet potato and butter beans if I'm aiming for a dish to keep us full all day long.

Heat a large lidded frying pan over a medium heat and spray it with a little oil.

Add the onion, red pepper and chilli to the pan and cook for a few minutes, stirring frequently.

Add the garlic and give it a good stir, then continue cooking until the pepper and onion start to brown.

Add the cumin, paprika and a pinch of salt to the pan, stir, then add the tomatoes and simmer for 10–12 minutes.

Using a large spoon, make four empty spaces in the pan for the eggs.

Crack the eggs into the gaps and cover the pan with a lid.

Cook for 7–10 minutes, or until the eggs are cooked.

Scatter over the feta, sprinkle over the chives and serve.

NOTE

If you've got an ovenproof pan, that's even better – bake at 180°C fan/400°F/gas mark 6 for 7–10 minutes instead.

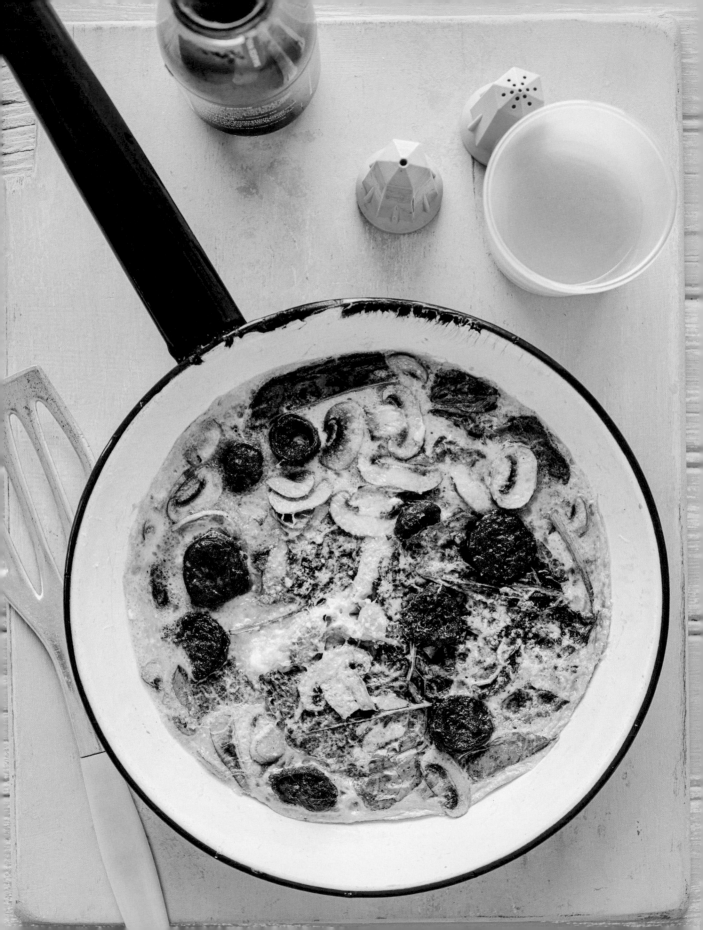

SPINACH, MUSHROOM & CHORIZO FRITTATA

SERVES: 1
PREP: 5 minutes
COOK: 15 minutes
CALORIES: 411

2 large eggs
40ml (1½fl oz) milk
40g (1½oz) chorizo, sliced
100g (3½oz) mushrooms, sliced
50g (1¾oz) baby spinach
10g (¼oz) Parmesan cheese, grated

You know how we're fans of the frittata here at Chubby Towers: it's one of those lunchbox staples that you can cook the night before in preparation for taking it into work the next day. And, if you're anything like us, you'll snaffle it all the night before and end up praying to the vending-machine gods next lunchtime.

I've always wanted to be one of those infuriating people who have an amazing lunch in the office – I used to work with someone who had a fancy bento box from which she would pull all manner of delicious-looking things. I was incredibly jealous: all I would have was a clingfilmed sweaty cheese and ham sandwich that had been in my bag since I started puberty. If you're the type who has the control to not eat their lunch at 9.03 a.m. *and* spend the evening before studiously preparing your lunchtime feast, then more power to your elbow.

You'll forgive me, of course, if I spend my spare time trying to throw staples into your coffee, yes?

Preheat the grill to medium-high.

Beat the eggs and milk together in a bowl and set aside.

Heat an 18cm (7 inch) frying pan over a medium heat and add the chorizo. Fry for a few minutes, then add the mushrooms. Cover the pan with a lid and cook until the mushrooms have softened, stirring occasionally.

Add the spinach to the pan and cook until wilted.

Add the egg mixture and cook until firm.

Sprinkle the Parmesan on top and transfer to the grill for a few minutes, until the cheese has browned.

BLACK FOREST SMOOTHIE

MAKES: 1
PREP: 5 minutes
COOK: 0 minutes
CALORIES: 277
DIET: VEG/GF

We have popped this recipe in as a bit of a gamble: we love smoothies, but also know that they are controversial among slimmers. Some people say it's a lot of sugar to have in one go, but we say that's a load of nonsense. One smoothie isn't going to totally wreck your diet. The old adage of 'you wouldn't eat all that fruit at once' just doesn't apply here: if you can't manage a few cherries and a bit of yoghurt, then you're clearly a sparrow.

The Black Forest theme makes me think of my nana, mentioned extensively in the last book. A Black Forest gâteau – thawed gently on the outside, as frozen as the polar ice-caps in the middle – would be plonked on the table after Sunday dinner. While she would have no time for such newfangled things as a smoothie (Dorothy was very much two slices of bread, two tubs of butter for breakfast), I had to tip her a wink somewhere in here.

This makes enough for one large glass of smoothie, but do scale as appropriate. I like a smoothie that is so thick it makes my cheeks suck in like I'm chewing a lemon, but if you prefer it thinner, just add some milk.

250g (9oz) fat-free natural
   yoghurt
100g (3½oz) frozen pitted sweet
   cherries
1 small banana
1 tsp good-quality cocoa powder
optional: squirty cream, a glacé
   cherry, chocolate shavings

Preheat the oven to 180°C fan/400°F/gas mark 6 and dig out a power-sander, you'll need it later.

I mean, clearly not, but we needed something to fill out the method.

Blend the yoghurt, cherries, banana and cocoa powder until as thick as a whale-egg omelette.

Thin with milk if you need to.

Top with squirty cream, a glacé cherry and chocolate shavings, if you're fancy.

NOTES

Smoothies freeze surprisingly well – if you find yourself at a loose end on a Sunday, you could triple the ingredients above, make enough for six smoothies and freeze them in mason jars for the week ahead.

Alternatively, if you pour the smoothie into ice-lolly moulds, you have a quick snack to grab when things are getting steamy.

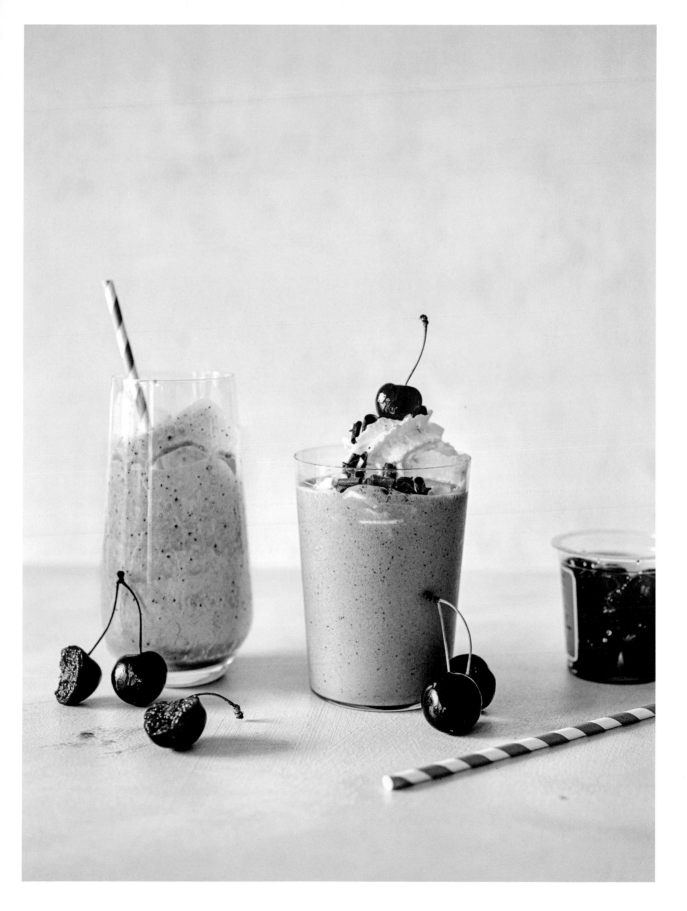

TURKISH POACHED EGGS

SERVES: 4
PREP: 5 minutes
COOK: 15 minutes
CALORIES: 321
DIET: VEG/GF

Trust us – this is beautiful. In Turkey it's called *cılbır* and it's a perfect snack or lunch! Also fantastic hangover food!

A poached egg is a thing of beauty – a friend of mine disagrees and calls anyone who orders them an absolute and utter sod, but it's probably years of serving them to people with faces like thunder in a roadside café that is colouring his view.

A note of caution, however: we previously recommended microwaving your poached egg. You can absolutely do this, but you must be ever so careful when handling the egg afterwards. Recently I, in my morning fog, was merrily making Paul's breakfast when I picked the egg up, only for the little bugger to betray me by blowing up in my face. Imagine having to go to A&E and explain your injuries were caused by an egg: mortifying. Plus, our kitchen ceiling now looks like it's covered in Artex – neither of us are tall enough to clean it.

Ah well. Live and learn. Caution in all things, people.

600g (1lb 5oz) fat-free Greek
   yoghurt
4 cloves of garlic, crushed
a pinch of salt
40g (1½oz) butter
1 tbsp dried chilli flakes
8 eggs

In a bowl, whisk together the yoghurt, garlic and a pinch of salt, and set aside (at room temperature).

Gently melt the butter in a small saucepan and add the chilli flakes, then keep warm.

Fill a large pan with water and bring to the boil, then reduce to a simmer.

Crack an egg into a small bowl, carefully pour into the water and repeat with the remaining eggs. Cook for 3–4 minutes. Remove with a slotted spoon and drain on a tea towel.

Divide the yoghurt among four plates and top with 2 eggs each. Drizzle over the butter.

NOTES

The yoghurt mix tastes best when it comes up to room temperature. Once you've mixed it, cover it and leave it out on the side while you make the rest.

Flatbreads are perfect for dipping into the eggs though make sure they're gluten-free if that's one of your dietary requirements.

SMART SWAP

You could use reduced-fat spread if you wish, but butter really does make it taste so much nicer (and it's not very much!).

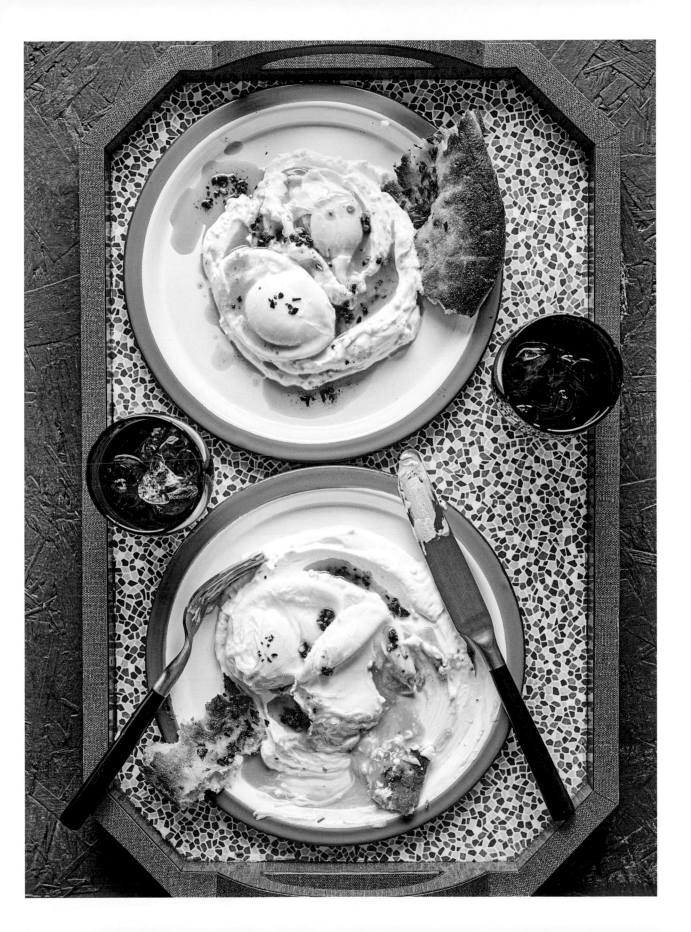

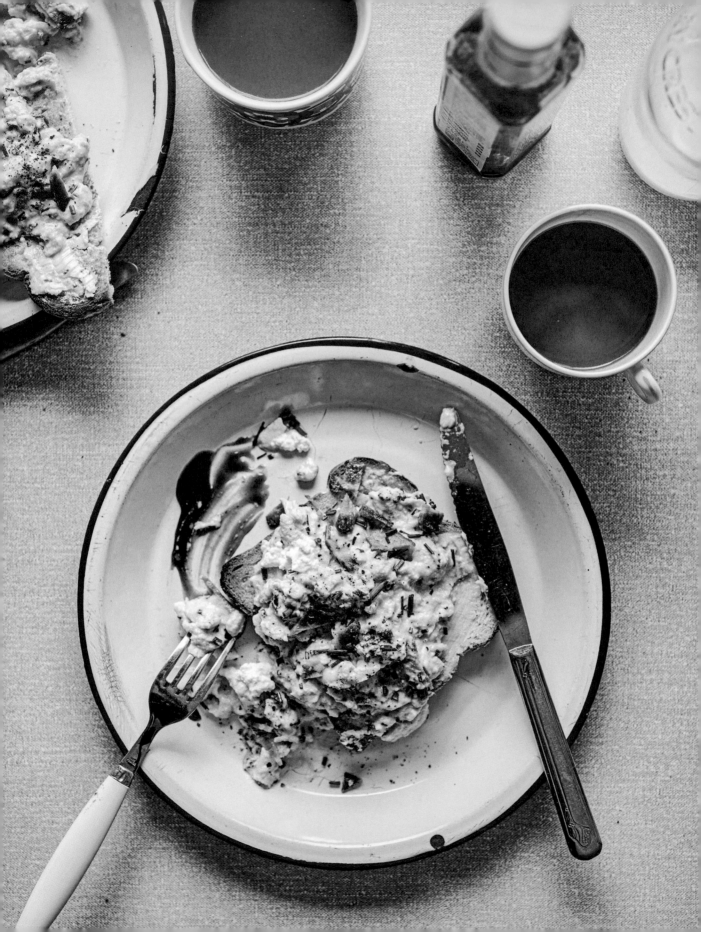

GREEN EGGS & FAM

SERVES: 4
PREP: 5 minutes
COOK: 10 minutes
CALORIES: 400

I can't pretend to know why Paul decided to call this recipe 'and fam' rather than ham: I think he's trying to be 'street'. That would work if he was the rough-hewn tart-with-a-heart I inherited thirteen years ago, but years of living with me and my fancy ways have softened his edges ever so much. That's my polite way of saying he's perfectly spherical.

When people meet us they always expect me to be the 'rough one' because I'm from Newcastle and have a face that suggests I live for a meat raffle in a flat-roof social club. They're always perfectly surprised by my impeccable manners, faultless modesty and clipped, terribly posh voice. Indeed, an *acquaintance* of mine has often threatened to call Trading Standards because he expected me to sound like Jimmy Nail when we met and instead got my lawyer-ish voice reading out a list of his shortcomings. Paul and I did once recreate the paintballing accident scene from *Byker Grove* in spectacular fashion, but modesty and the book's age-rating prevent me from sharing the details.

Anyway: it's all an act. I was 'asked' when I started my job to refine my telephone voice because apparently clients don't like to discuss sensitive legal matters with someone who sounds as though they're selling strawberries from a windswept market stall. Pah. I'd give it all up for a 'canny bag of Tudor', though …

4 rashers of bacon
8 eggs
2 tbsp chopped fresh chives
200g (7oz) ricotta
4 slices of toast

Spray a frying pan with a little oil and place it over a high heat. Add the bacon and cook until crispy, then remove to a plate and chop roughly. Place the pan back over a low heat.

Whisk together the eggs and chives and pour into the pan, sprinkling in the bacon. Mix constantly with a wooden spoon for about a minute, until you get firm bits of egg along with some runny.

Remove from the heat and fold in the ricotta – don't bother being too neat about this, big chunks are fine.

Arrange over the toast and serve.

NOTE

We quite like this with a bit of brown sauce and a grind of black pepper. You do you though.

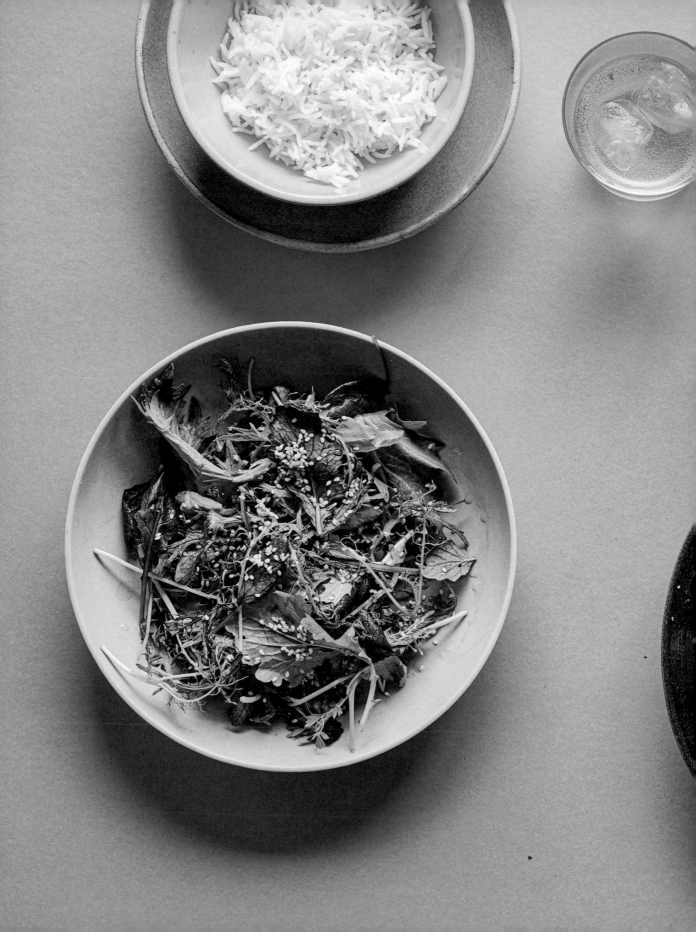

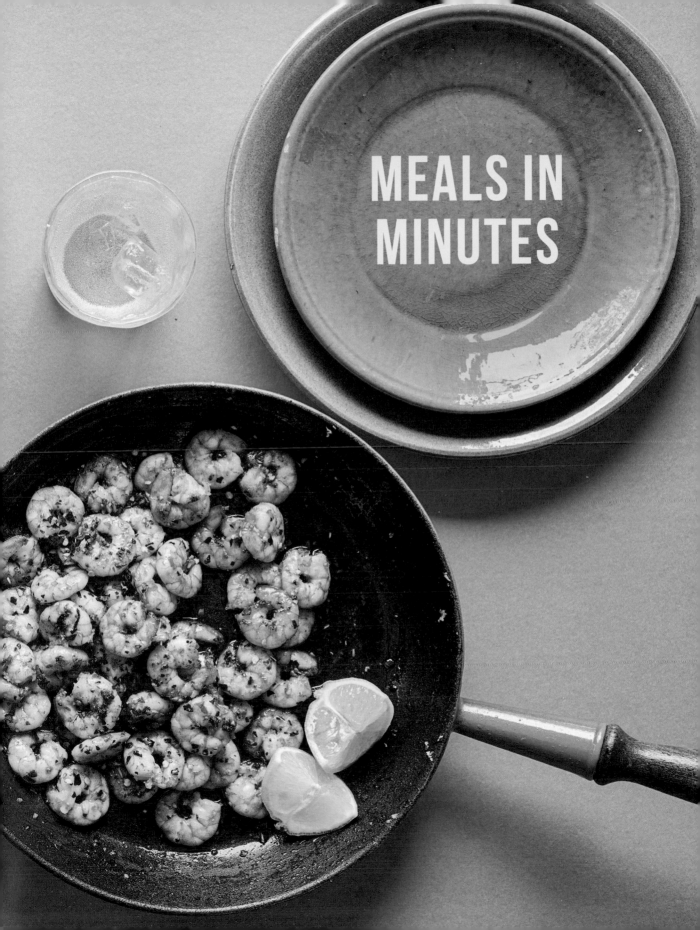

MEALS IN
MINUTES

ROSEMARY-CRUSTED LAMB STEAKS

SERVES: 4
PREP: 5 minutes
COOK: 10 minutes
CALORIES: 400

We always struggle a bit with lamb recipes. See, despite having a heart as black as pitch and a soul that can never be saved, I also have a conscience. And, let's be fair, lambs are bloody adorable. I know I'm a colossal hypocrite on this vegetarian/meat-eating stance, but shall we all agree to disagree and move on?

I've actually done my bit to bring lambs into the world: growing up in the country wasn't just passionate summer trysts with the local country boys, you know. I was called into action one night to assist with lambing and I need to tell you, it was horrifying. I was shown what to do, given gentle encouragement and then told to hurry the fuck up because there was no time for me to clip my nails and shriek. In the end, I reached in, gently moved the lamb's head and feet into place and boom, out it came.

I'm not saying I'm a hero here, but given that it was like putting my hand into a Wellington boot stuffed with wafer-thin ham and hot mayonnaise, I deserve a medal.

And Christ, if that doesn't make you want to try the recipe, what will? I promise you this is delicious, but I couldn't spare the analogy!

50g (1¾oz) fresh parsley
2 tbsp fresh rosemary
1 clove of garlic
2 tbsp grated Parmesan cheese
60g (2¼oz) breadcrumbs
4 tsp olive oil
1 egg, beaten
4 lamb steaks

Put the parsley, rosemary, garlic, Parmesan, breadcrumbs and 3 teaspoons of the olive oil into a food processor and blitz to a pesto-like consistency.

Pour the beaten egg into a shallow dish and pour the pesto into another dish.

Gently dip each of the lamb steaks into the egg and then into the pesto.

Heat a large pan over a medium-high heat and add the remaining oil. Add the lamb in batches and cook for about 2 minutes on each side, then remove from the pan and leave to rest for 3–5 minutes.

Serve!

NOTE

We love these with some standard mash and broccoli, but you do what you like. They are cracking for a Sunday dinner!

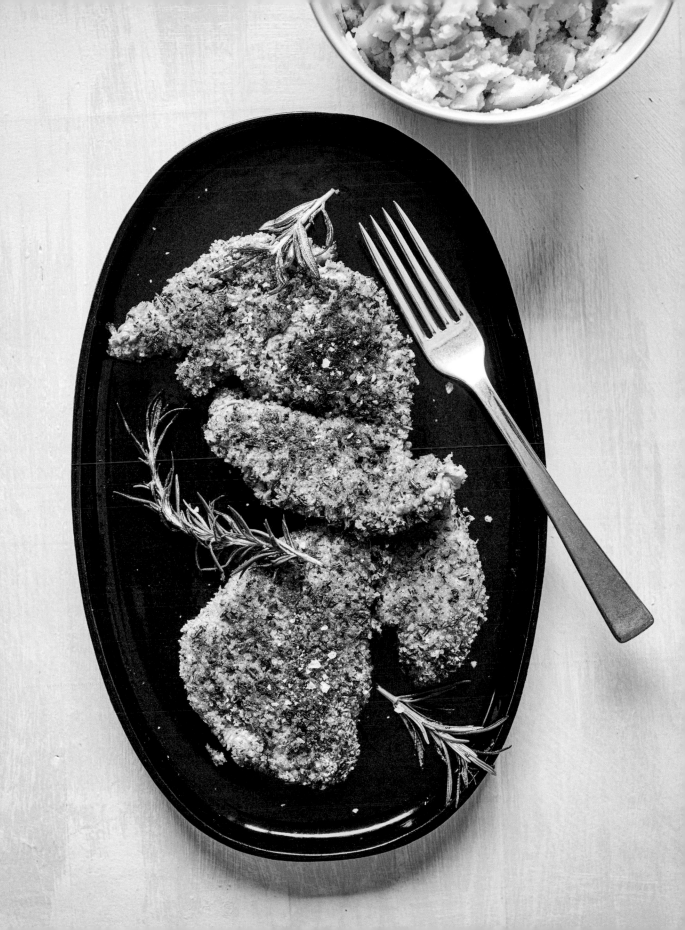

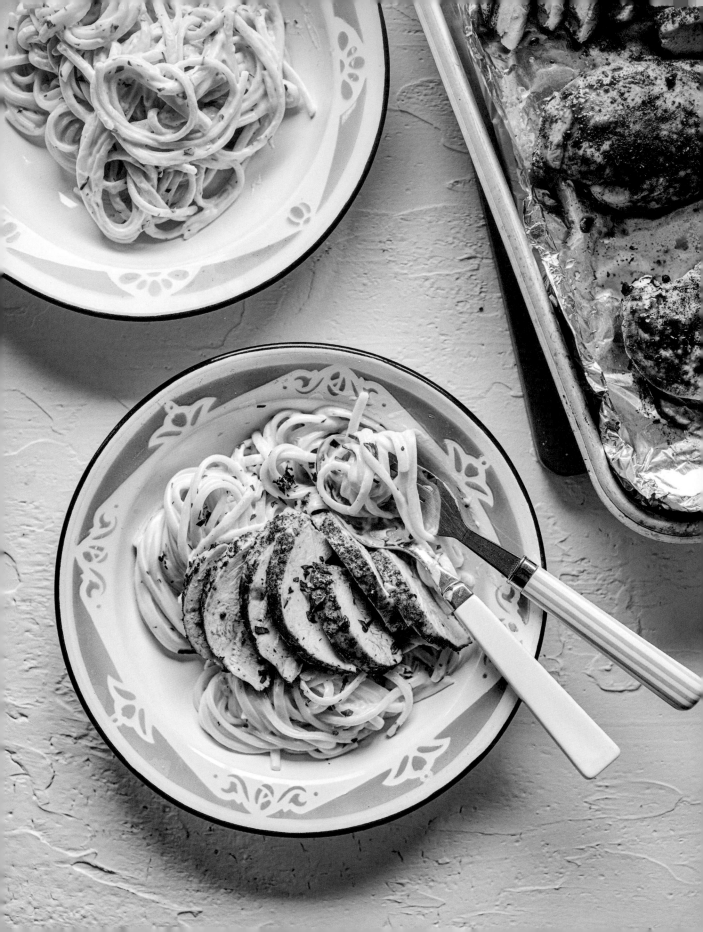

CHUBBY CHICKEN ALFREDO

SERVES: 4
PREP: 10 minutes
COOK: 20 minutes
CALORIES: 499

We bloody love a chicken alfredo here at Chubby Towers and are chuffed that we have managed to make a 'skinny' version. It's usually made with double cream and enough cheese to require a defibrillator on standby, but this lighter version works ever so well.

That chubby in the title is a nasty business, though – we do like to scatter chubby about, though we worry about the connotations. See, we could get away with it when we were young and podgy – it seemed cute and cuddly, like a dog given one too many treats. Now it seems ever so slightly misleading, like a man's idea of eight inches. We've discussed rebranding but it's so bedded in now that we can't.

Woe may be us, then, but this recipe will give you life. Go ahead.

4 skinless, boneless chicken breasts
1 tsp dried mixed herbs
½ tsp paprika
¼ tsp salt, plus an extra pinch
¼ tsp black pepper
250g (9oz) spaghetti
2 cloves of garlic, crushed
250ml (9fl oz) semi-skimmed milk
1 tbsp plain flour
4 tbsp light cream cheese
20g (¾oz) Parmesan cheese, grated
a pinch of grated nutmeg
2 tbsp chopped fresh parsley

Preheat the oven to 220°C fan/450°F/gas mark 9.

Put the chicken breasts on a baking sheet. Mix together the mixed herbs, paprika, salt and pepper and rub into the chicken breasts. Cook in the oven for 15–20 minutes.

Meanwhile, bring a large pan of salted water to the boil. Cook the spaghetti according to the packet instructions, then drain.

While the spaghetti and chicken are cooking, heat a saucepan over a medium heat and spray it with a little oil. Add the garlic and cook for 1 minute.

Add the milk and flour and stir continuously until smooth. Once thickened, remove the pan from the heat and add the soft cheese, Parmesan, nutmeg and a pinch of salt.

Toss the drained pasta with the sauce and divide between four plates.

Remove the chicken from the oven, slice, then top each plate of pasta with a sliced chicken breast and sprinkle over the parsley.

NOTE

If you set the spaghetti, chicken and sauce away at the same time, they'll all finish together, so it's worth spending a few minutes at the start prepping everything.

PRAWN COCKTAIL WRAPS

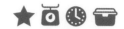

SERVES: 4
PREP: 10 minutes
COOK: 0 minutes
CALORIES: 230

I have a confession. Now, it's nothing as exciting as revealing where Shergar buggered off to or admitting to my part in the Brinks-Mat robbery (which in itself would have been quite a feat considering I was merely a twinkle in my dad's wandering eye at that point). No, it's far more sedate. I fibbed in the last book when I said I didn't like prawns. I know, I'm a horror – if you're thinking of setting up a Twitter hate campaign, as is *de rigueur* these days, may I suggest #hardcoreprawn as a hashtag?

In my defence, such as it is, I do vehemently dislike those tiny wee prawns you get served in a pot of pink sauce at the seaside. But I understand that those mealy little worms are as close to prawns as I am to settling down with a lovely wife and raising some children. This recipe takes those fancy big buggers you buy cooked and mixes them with avocado in a wrap that brings to mind every seventies dinner you ever attended.

Only this time, leave your keys in your pocket.

1 avocado
1 tbsp lemon juice
150g (5½oz) cooked and peeled
    prawns
1 tbsp extra-light mayonnaise
1 tbsp tomato ketchup
1 little gem lettuce
½ cucumber
4 wholemeal wraps

Halve the avocado, scoop out the flesh, and mash in a bowl with the lemon juice.

Next, gently mix together the prawns, mayonnaise and tomato ketchup and set aside.

Wash and roughly chop the lettuce, and set aside.

Using a peeler (or even better, a julienne slicer), slice the cucumber into ribbons.

Spread the avocado over one-quarter of each wrap, top with the prawns, lettuce and cucumber, then turn up the bottom edge and roll to assemble the wrap.

NOTE

If you're feeling fancy, add a pinch of smoked paprika to the mix.

SMART SWAP

We're big fans of chunky jumbo prawns in this, but you use whatever you like!

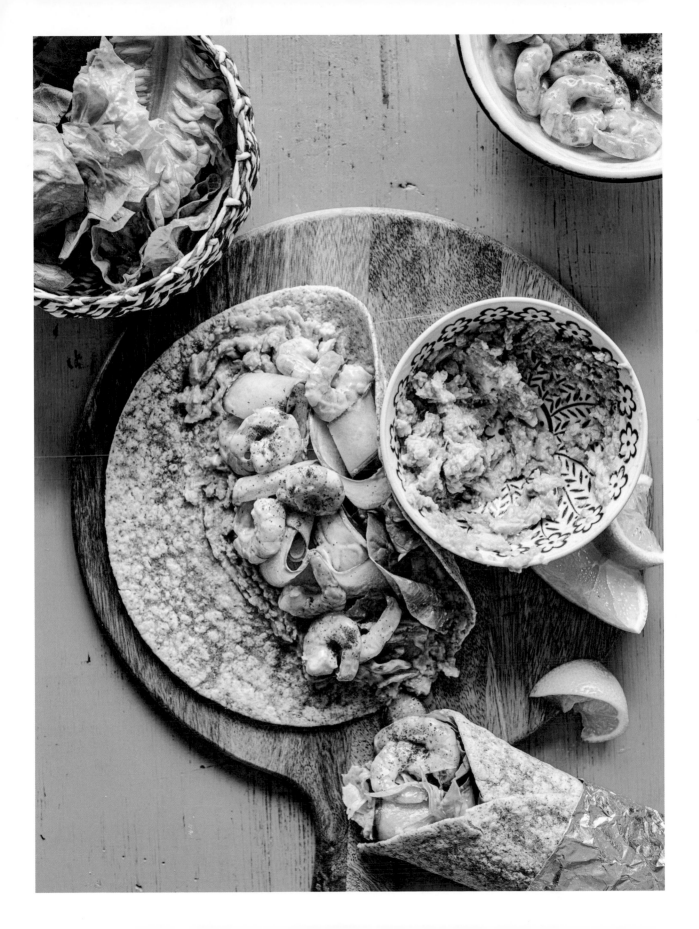

CHORIZO & BROCCOLI GNOCCHI

SERVES: 4
PREP: 15 minutes
COOK: 15 minutes
CALORIES: 478

150g (5½oz) chorizo, diced
3 cloves of garlic, crushed
1 head of broccoli, chopped into
  small florets
125ml (4fl oz) chicken stock
200g (7oz) extra-light soft cheese
4 sun-dried tomatoes, finely
  chopped
½ tbsp Dijon mustard
120g (4½oz) baby spinach
500g (1lb 2oz) gnocchi
40g (1½oz) Parmesan cheese,
  grated

We have spoken about our love affairs with both chorizo and gnocchi before, so I'll spare you a repeat, but we encourage you to give this dish a try.

One thing I will say: please don't do what we used to do and substitute gnocchi with new potatoes to try and save a few calories. You mustn't. While the dish would probably still work, the gnocchi acts as a flavour-hoover and you'll be rewarded with slightly crunchy bursts of yum in this.

This does sit well in the fridge for leftovers, but please, none of us got to the point where we were breathless sliding our shoes on because we left our plates unfinished.

Place a large frying pan over a medium-high heat. Add the chorizo and garlic and cook for 1 minute. Add the broccoli and cook for another 3–4 minutes.

Stir in the stock and simmer for 2 minutes, then reduce the heat to medium. Add the soft cheese, sun-dried tomatoes and mustard, and mix well.

Stir in the spinach and reduce the heat again to low.

Bring a large saucepan of water to the boil and add the gnocchi. Cook according to the packet instructions, then drain (reserving half a mug of the cooking water).

Add the gnocchi to the frying pan and stir gently, adding some of the reserved cooking water if the mix seems a little thick or dry.

Serve sprinkled with the Parmesan.

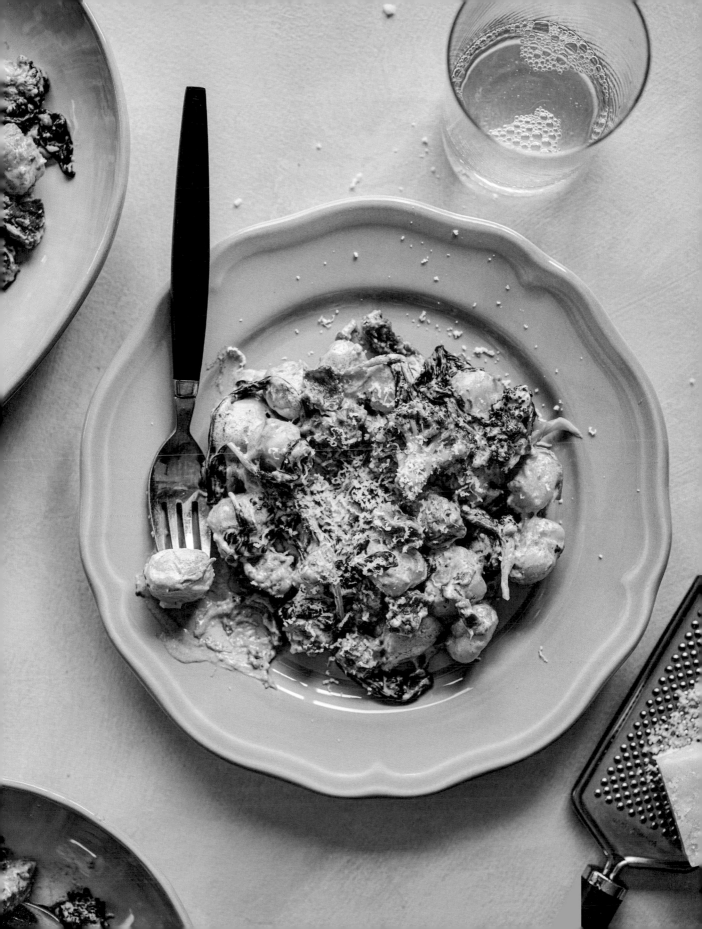

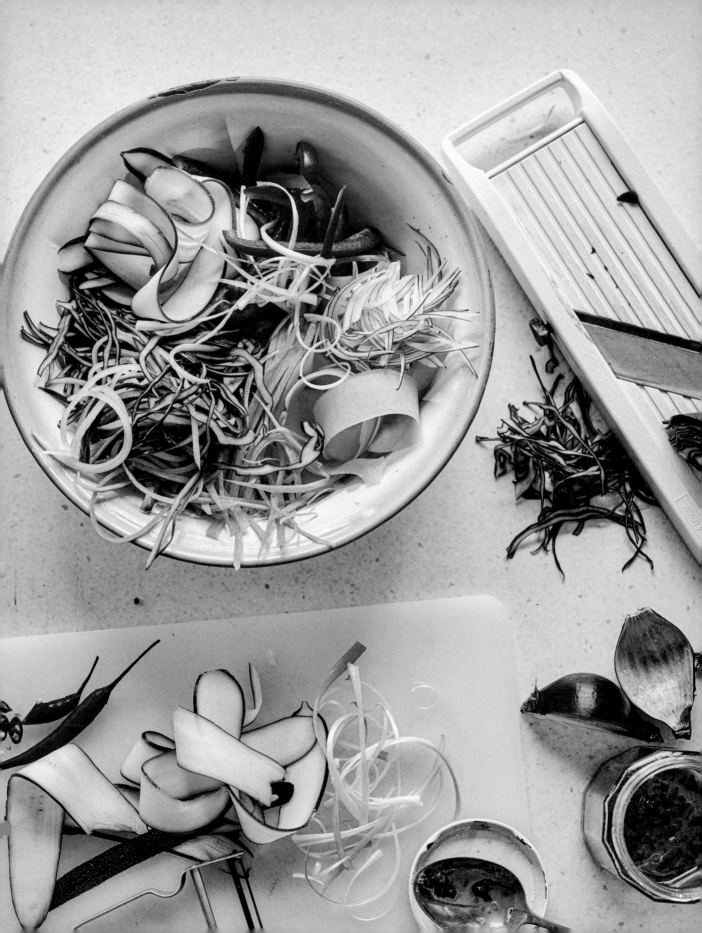

PICK 'N' MIX SALAD

SERVES: 4
PREP: 20 minutes
COOK: 0 minutes
CALORIES: 106
DIET: VEG/V/GF/DF

This recipe is a case of throwing together whatever you can get your hands on (that doesn't include slipping chips in there, you little terror). We have included two separate dressings – both add zing but only one of them will trouble your nethers if you're not a fan of heat. The salad ingredients are meant as a 'suggestion' – add whatever you like, leave out what doesn't thrill you. Depending on how many vegetables you use, this can serve as many as you like.

We beg of you, though: invest in a good julienne peeler or at least go steady with your knife or mandolin slicer. We have lost so many bits of fingers that these days a salad isn't complete unless I'm picking thumbnail from my teeth two days later.

Pick from:

1 large carrot, peeled and julienned

1 small butternut squash, peeled into ribbons

1 small red cabbage, halved and very finely sliced

a bunch of spring onions, root cut off, then sliced lengthways to make ribbons

1 large red pepper, finely sliced

1 small red onion, finely sliced

1 small cucumber, julienned into ribbons, avoiding the seeds

1 large courgette (if you can get yellow courgettes, even better), peeled into ribbons

a handful of spinach, rolled into a cigar shape and then finely chopped

Mild dressing

equal parts apple cider vinegar (see below) to olive oil, with a pinch of salt and pepper

Hot dressing

1 small red chilli (deseeded), chopped very fine and mixed with 2 tablespoons of lime juice, 1 tablespoon of olive oil and a pinch of sugar

Wash all your vegetables – under the tap will do, we're not expecting you to throw them in with your unmentionables.

Assemble, but do read the notes below.

NOTES

This is a 'dress and eat' salad – don't dress it unless you plan to eat it – you want it crunchy!

Prepare the courgette and spinach last – the rest of the vegetables stand up to being left for a while, but the courgette can brown and the spinach will wilt.

If a strong onion taste just doesn't chive with you (boom!), when you finely slice the red onion, pop it into some apple cider vinegar for 20 minutes to take the sting away.

Don't throw away that vinegar either – it's great on chips!

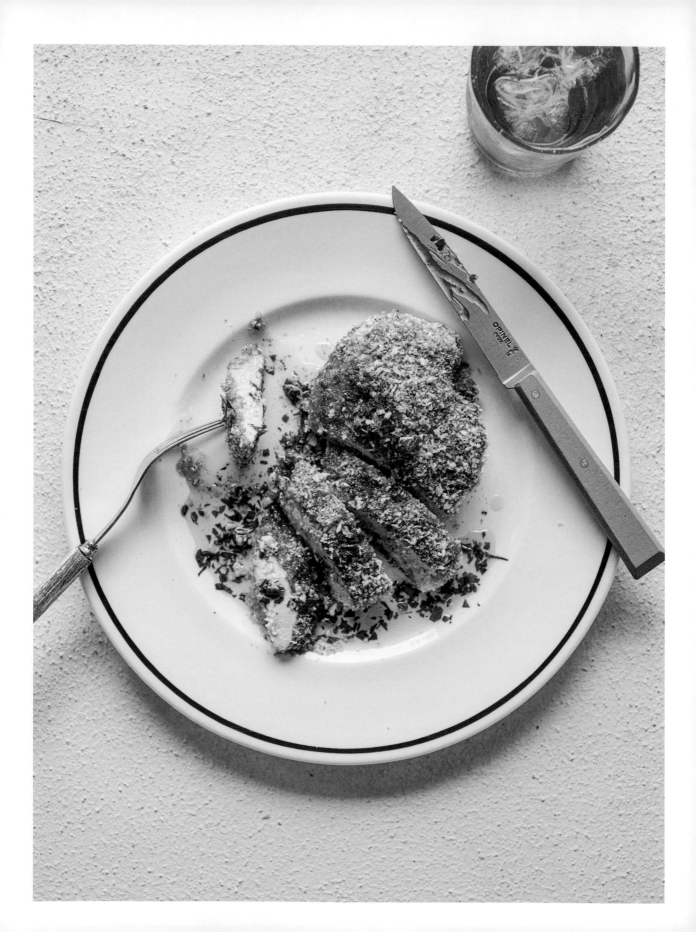

LAZY CHICKEN KIEVS

SERVES: 4
PREP: 5 minutes
COOK: 25 minutes
CALORIES: 368

We're calling these lazy chicken Kievs because 'inside out Kiev' sounds like a handsome lad I had over once. Goodness me, he was accommodating.

I have a plea for you, though: you might be tempted to skip this recipe due to the butter, but it's the garlic butter that makes the dish. If you genuinely can't treat yourself, you can swap out the butter for some extra-light soft cheese – just loosen it up over a low heat and pour over.

Incidentally, if you had a bit of time, it's no trouble at all to turn this into a proper chicken Kiev – just cut a gash in the side of the chicken breast, snicker to yourself at the word gash, make your garlic butter and leave to cool, then slip it in there. If you have cocktail sticks, use them to hold the chicken shut while you cook it.

Oh! And yet another fabulous tip – mop up any remnants in the pan with some grilled bread of choice for delicious garlicky goodness. I know, we spoil you.

4 skinless, boneless chicken breasts
2 eggs, beaten
25g (1oz) panko breadcrumbs
4 cloves of garlic, crushed
75g (2½oz) butter
2 tbsp finely chopped fresh parsley

Preheat the oven to 180°C fan/400°F/gas mark 6.

Dip each chicken breast in the beaten egg, then roll them in the breadcrumbs until well coated.

Place the chicken on a baking tray lined with greaseproof paper and bake in the oven for 20–25 minutes.

Meanwhile, spray a small saucepan with a little oil and place it over a medium heat.

Add the garlic and stir around the pan for a minute or two.

Add the butter and stir until melted, then add the parsley and stir to mix.

Serve the chicken and drizzle the butter sauce over the top.

SMART SWAP

Can't get panko breadcrumbs?
Any breadcrumbs will do!

HONEY & CHILLI GARLIC PRAWNS

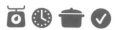

SERVES: 4
PREP: 5 minutes
COOK: 10 minutes
CALORIES: 105
DIET: DF

I happened across these spicy little buggers at one of the rare networking events I was forced to go to (happily attended) through work last year. Because, honestly, what better things to cram in your gob while you're trying to make strained conversation with someone you'll never meet again than honking garlic prawns? Name me a better incentive to 'call you later' than a fish and garlic combination. I'll wait.

OK, I've waited long enough. Don't let my intro put you off – these really are quite something, and I'm just jaundiced because I can't bear networking events. I'm a Chatty Cathy at the best of times, but I struggle ever so with large crowds because I can never remember important details like names and job titles. Someone could ask me to write my name on the sign-in sheet and I'll be so overcome with lethologica and angst that I'll cheerfully announce that I've shat myself and must leave immediately. It's truly exhausting being so highly strung, I promise you.

If you're not a fan of prawns, swap them out for little tiny cocktail sausages. Or massive sausages, you size-shaming terror.

500g (1lb 2oz) cooked and
    peeled king prawns
4 cloves of garlic, crushed
2 tsp dried chilli flakes
5cm (2 inches) ginger,
    finely grated
1 tsp honey
1 tsp light or dark soy sauce
½ a lemon

Gently toss the prawns with the garlic and chilli flakes.

Spray a large frying pan with a little oil and place it over a medium heat. Add the prawns and cook for 2–3 minutes, stirring constantly, then scoop them out of the pan and set aside.

Reduce the heat to low and add the ginger, stir well, then add the honey. Add 120ml (4fl oz) of water and stir, deglazing the pan if necessary. Add the soy sauce and bring to a simmer.

Put the prawns back into the pan and cook for 1 minute.

Squeeze over the lemon juice and serve.

NOTE
Serve with a nice green salad.

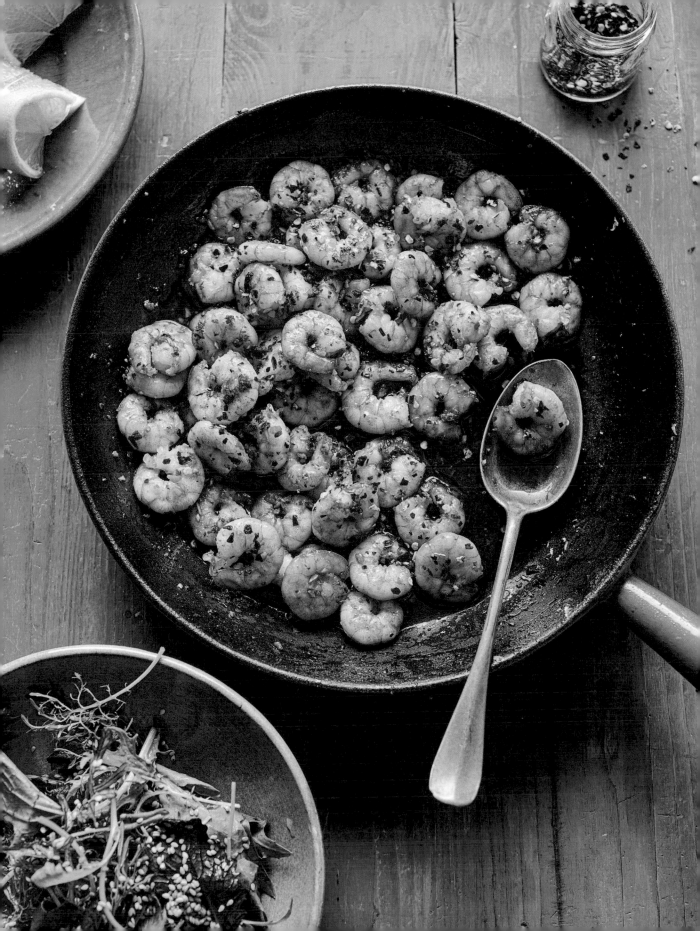

BACON & BLUE CHEESE SALAD

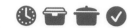

SERVES: 4
PREP: 10 minutes
COOK: 5 minutes
CALORIES: 266
DIET: GF

As mentioned in the notes below, if you're not a fan of blue cheese, we can understand, and you can swap it out for something milder (though not Swiss cheese: we can't bear their holier-than-thou stance). But if I may encourage you to keep trying with blue cheese, one day it'll just work for you – it'll go from smelling like someone's died to being heaven itself.

Note – when Paul gave me this recipe, he told me not to repeat my cringeworthy entry from the last book where I littered a recipe intro with puns. Don't use cheese puns? Edam, how dairy! I said, you Gouda be kidding! I've matured since then! Telling me how to write – I Camembert it!

OK, buckle in, folks. No apologies given. Ricotta get through this.

6 bacon medallions, diced
600g (1lb 5oz) green leaves
(see smart swaps)
2 celery stalks, finely sliced
4 spring onions, finely sliced
1 tbsp finely chopped fresh
parsley
125g (4½oz) fat-free Greek
yoghurt
2 tsp cider vinegar
¼ tsp salt
¼ tsp black pepper
100g (3½oz) blue cheese,
crumbled (see smart swaps)
2 tbsp sliced chives

Spray a frying pan with a little oil and place it over a high heat. Add the bacon and cook until crispy, then set aside.

Mix together the green leaves, celery, spring onions and parsley and serve on plates, topped with the bacon.

Mix together the Greek yoghurt, cider vinegar, salt, pepper and blue cheese and drizzle over the salad.

Sprinkle over the sliced chives and serve.

SMART SWAPS

Use whatever green leaves you like in this – we like to use a combination of lettuce, baby spinach and rocket to give a bit of zing, but it's really up to you!

We tend to use the milder Danish Blue or Gorgonzola in this, but stronger cheeses like Stilton are grand too. If you're not a fan of blue cheese, soft goat's cheese also goes well.

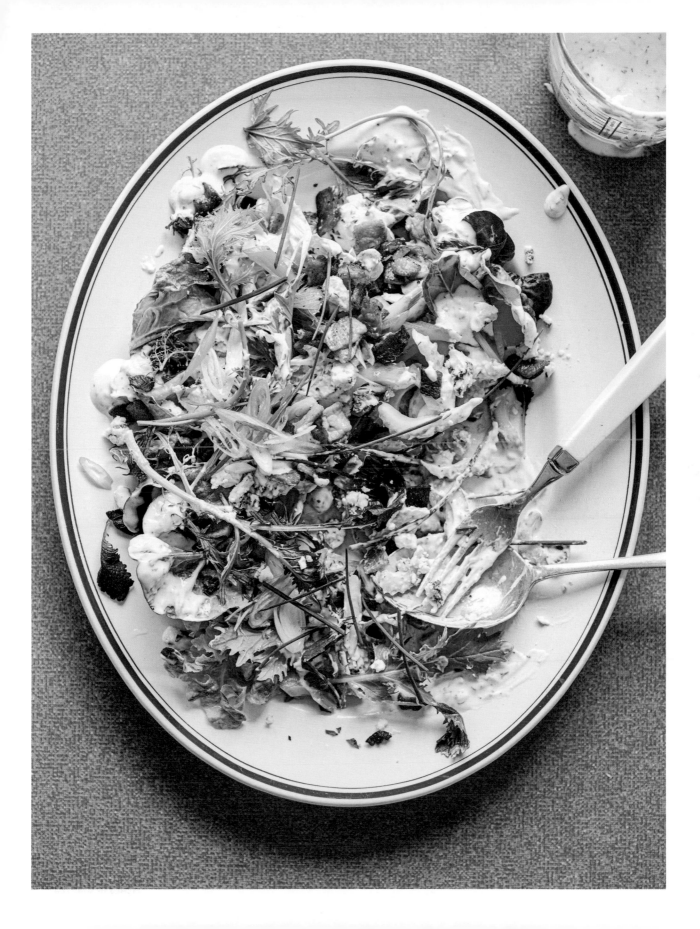

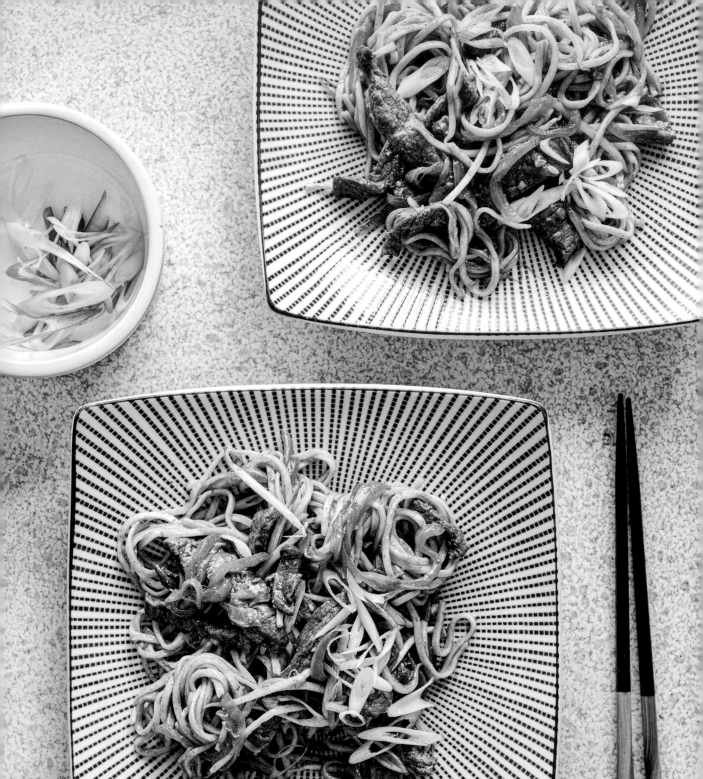

QUICK BEEFY NOODLES

SERVES: 4
PREP: 5 minutes
COOK: 10 minutes
CALORIES: 486
DIET: DF

One of our favourite quick dishes, this: it's almost like a chow mein, but a little saucier. Paul can throw this together in a matter of moments with his professional yet slipshod approach in the kitchen.

I always appreciate a quick dinner at Chubby Towers because it means less time listening to Paul's abysmal taste in music blaring through the speakers. We've covered his bewildering love of Tracy Chapman many times over the years, but even when he branches out into new music, he just ends up playing the same songs over and over. And lord: the singing. I'm not saying he's out of tune, but there's been several times I've had to mince in to check he hasn't shut the cat in the oven.

I, on the other hand, can sing beautifully, and I'll ignore anyone who winces at me as I reach for the high notes. I will say this: when we're singing together, we have a great time, with many a road-trip spent absolutely slaughtering the classics and getting spittle on the windscreen as we go.

Curious about our couple song, by the way? I can't imagine you are, but this is my book and you're captive: it's 'Sunshine' by River Matthews.

Well, it was never gonna be bloody Coldplay, was it?

300g (10½oz) dried noodles
1 tbsp dark soy sauce
1 tbsp oyster sauce
1 tbsp hoisin sauce
1 tbsp cider vinegar
2 tsp sesame oil
½ onion, sliced
3 cloves of garlic, crushed
400g (14oz) stir-fry beef strips
100g (3½oz) beansprouts
2 spring onions, sliced

Cook the noodles according to the packet instructions, then drain and set aside.

Meanwhile, mix together the soy sauce, oyster sauce, hoisin sauce, cider vinegar and sesame oil.

Heat a large frying pan over a high heat and spray it with a little oil. Add the onion and garlic and cook for a few minutes. Add the beef and cook until just a little pink remains.

Add the sauce and cook for another 2–3 minutes.

Add the beansprouts and cook for another minute until steaming hot.

Add the cooked noodles and stir until everything is coated.

Serve, sprinkled with the spring onions.

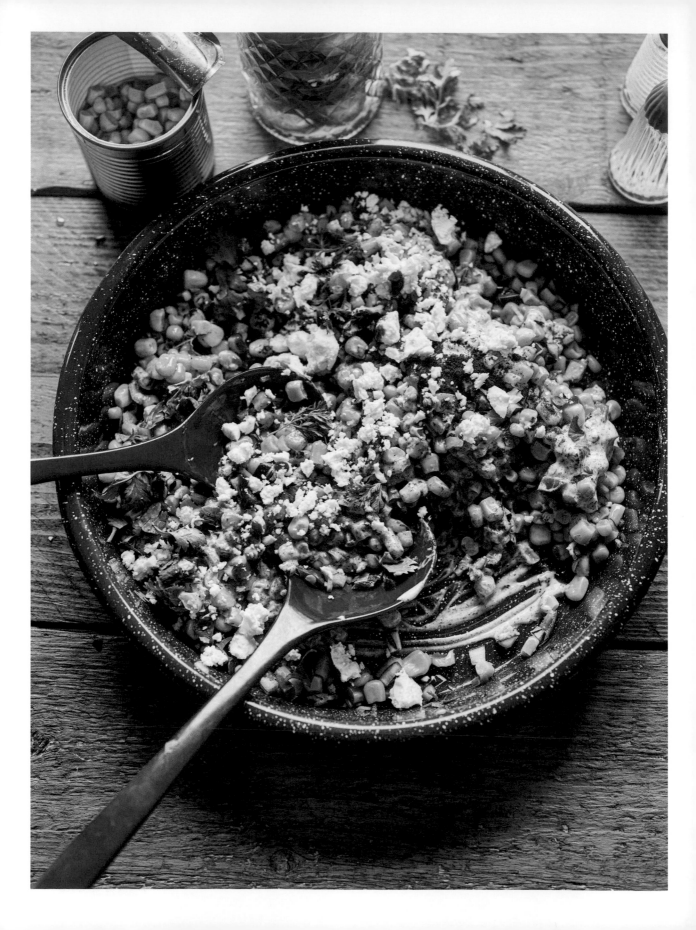

MEXICAN CORN SALAD

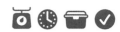

SERVES: 4
PREP: 10 minutes
COOK: 0 minutes
CALORIES: 172
DIET: VEG (check feta is vegetarian friendly)

Mexican food is quite possibly my favourite food in the world, though I maintain I've only had excellent Mexican food once before. Naturally, that was in Albufeira where we had a fabulous holiday a couple of years ago.

I also suffered one of the most painful moments of my life in a waterpark. Now, listen, we adore waterparks, but fat hairy men do not do well in them. Let me explain in sequence.

Being fat means you either go hurtling down the slides at such a lick that you come out at the bottom like a launched torpedo and smack your ankles off the bottom of the pool, or, it's a slow, squeaky descent to the bottom with water pooling behind your back-boobs.

Being hairy, especially on your back, means every time you ricochet over a seam in the slide you lose half your pelt – and that bloody hurts! Paul is as hairless as the day he was born and so goes scooting down the slides like an oiled otter.

Finally, those slides where you hurl yourself forward, landing on the mat that carries you down? Aye, grand until you land on your own testicles, which are making a bid for freedom via your ankles in the sweltering heat. That's exactly what I did, and is why I spent the rest of the holiday walking like I'd shat myself.

On that note, CORN!

350g (12oz) tinned sweetcorn
   (drained weight)
1 tbsp butter, melted
1 red onion, finely diced
30g (1oz) reduced-fat feta cheese,
   crumbled
2 tbsp light mayonnaise
1 tbsp lemon juice
1 tsp dried chilli flakes
1 tbsp sliced jalapeños, diced
a few drops of sriracha
2 tsp paprika
a handful of fresh coriander
   leaves, chopped

Chuck everything into a bowl and mix well.

NOTE

This is champion as a lunch idea on its own, or as a side.

ITALIAN SAUSAGE CARBONARA

SERVES: 4
PREP: 10 minutes
COOK: 20 minutes
CALORIES: 347

Our carbonara is legendary in slimming circles. We seem to be the only ones out there who make a carbonara the way it ought to be made: with no bloody soft cheese or Quark involved. Carbonara should be as silky as a conman's whisper and that's the very end of it.

Over the years we've witnessed all sorts of excitingly awful combinations, like vanilla yoghurt used in Coronation chicken, and they'll moo 'It tastes just like the real thing!'. Aye, if the only way you've tasted the real thing is through your own fevered imagination.

We *have* taken an indulgence with this recipe by adding fennel seeds (more faces than the town clock, me), but it's to add an extra note of flavour. If you want to be as pure as the driven snow (and good luck with that, what with *your* record), you can leave out the sausages and fennel seeds.

250g (9oz) tagliatelle
30g (1oz) Parmesan cheese, grated
3 eggs
4 tsp dried parsley
½ tsp fennel seeds
4 low-fat sausages

Cook the tagliatelle according to the packet instructions, then drain (keeping aside half a mug of the cooking water).

In a bowl, whisk the Parmesan with the eggs and parsley, and set aside.

Meanwhile, crush the fennel seeds as best you can – a pestle and mortar are perfect for the job, or use the end of a rolling pin.

Squeeze the meat out of the sausages and discard the casings.

Heat a large frying pan over a medium-high heat and spray it with a little oil. Add the sausage meat to the pan with the crushed fennel seeds and cook for about 5–6 minutes, breaking it up with a spatula.

Add the drained pasta to the pan and spread it out well. Add 1 tablespoon of the reserved pasta cooking water to stop it drying out.

Pour over the egg mixture and toss well to combine.

Serve.

NOTE

If you can get fresh parsley, that's even better – you'll need about 5g (⅛oz).

SMART SWAPS

You can swap fennel for sage to make a sort of Lincolnshire sausage carbonara!

You can use vegetarian sausages if you're that way inclined. Though, be sure to use vegetarian Italian hard cheese instead as Parmesan cheese contains animal rennet.

Any pasta will do.

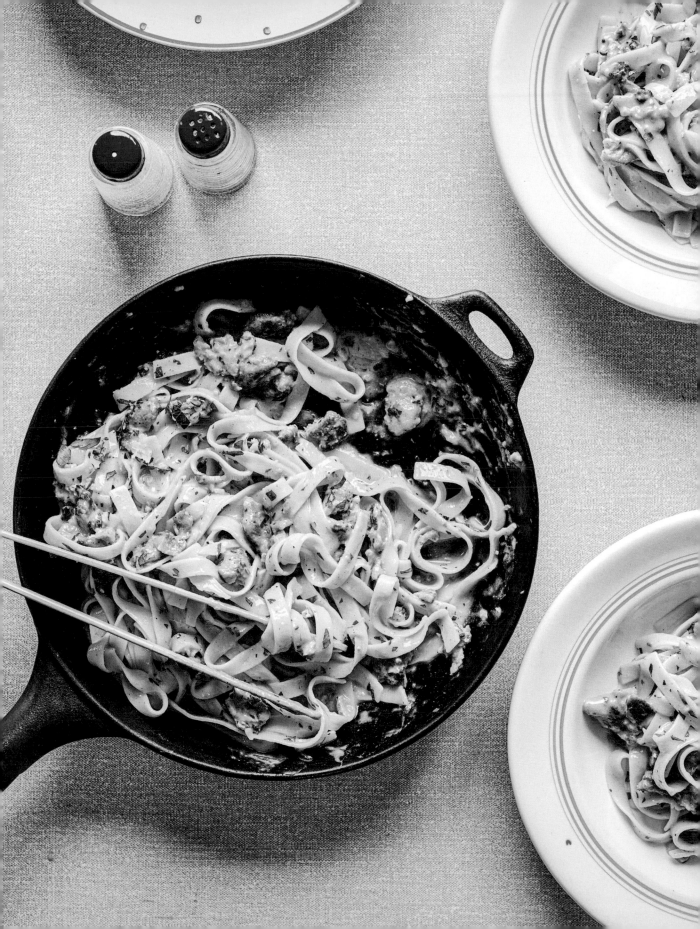

PAN-FRIED COD WITH A BUTTERY LEMON & HERB SAUCE

SERVES: 4
PREP: 5 minutes
COOK: 10 minutes
CALORIES: 219
DIET: GF

A recipe that makes me think of two things. First, my nana, who used to poach fish in milk, only she would set it away on a Tuesday morning so it was ready for her Sunday tea. This meant her house was absolutely honking of fish but any nasal distress paled in comparison to having my eardrums reduced to a fine mist via the medium of *Fifteen to One* being played at a volume akin to a jet engine taking off.

The second is the first and only time we've ever stayed at a B&B, where Paul was given this dish for supper. We can't cope with B&Bs – on paper, they're a great idea, but (admittedly based on this lone experience) in reality they're a fraught exercise in forced politeness and bewildering rules. A lady who had never known what it was to smile showed us to our room and then spent fifteen minutes telling us what we weren't to do. I've had more pleasurable rectal examinations. We went to bed at 9.30 p.m. purely out of worry we had upset her, and breakfast the next day was served with such anger and hostility that I had to check we hadn't just wandered into a stranger's home. Never again. Fish was good, though.

Of course, should any B&B owner want to host us and prove us wrong, get in touch. We promise not to leave pants everywhere.

4 skin-on, boneless cod fillets
40g (1½oz) butter
½ lemon
1 tsp dried parsley
1 tsp finely chopped fresh chives
1 tsp dried tarragon

Spray a large frying pan with a little oil and place it over a medium heat. Add the fish to the pan, skin side down, and cook for 2 minutes.

Add a few small chunks of butter around the fish and cook for another 1–2 minutes.

Gently turn the fish over and cook for another 3–4 minutes, then remove from the pan on to plates. Add the rest of the butter to the pan and stir until melted.

Squeeze the juice of the lemon into the pan (make sure to catch any pips!) and add the herbs. Stir well.

Spoon the butter sauce over the fish and serve.

NOTE

We love this with some new potatoes and broccoli, or chips if we're feeling grotty.

SMART SWAP

Any white fish will do! Haddock, pollock and hake are great alternatives. You can also use skinless fish if you prefer – just be careful when turning it.

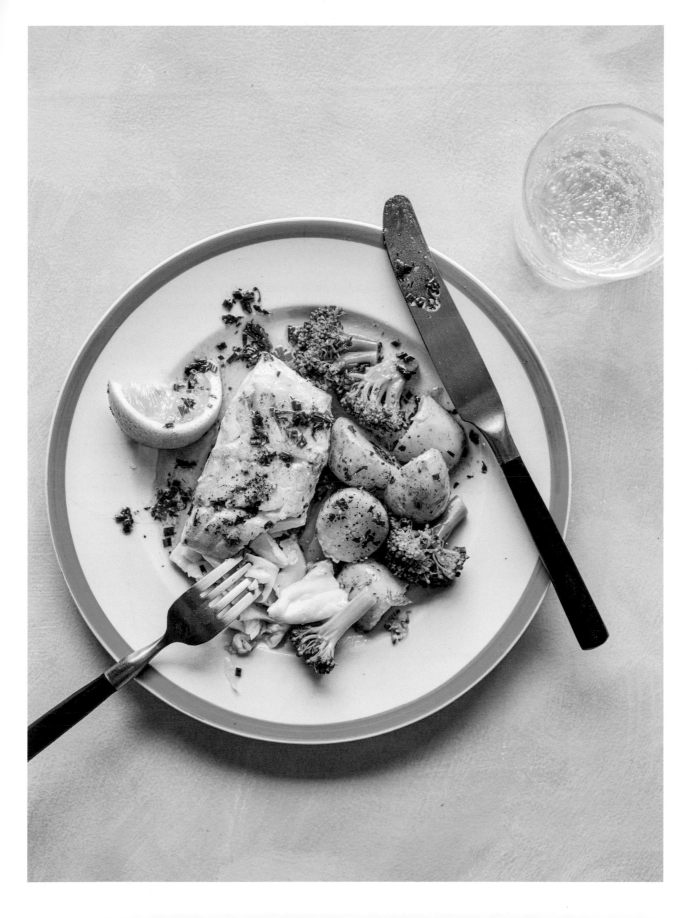

HONEY & GARLIC BEEF

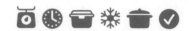

SERVES: 4
PREP: 10 minutes
COOK: 15 minutes
CALORIES: 300
DIET: GF

Sometimes you just want something sweet and sticky and this is the perfect meal for those occasions – it only takes a few minutes of bustling to throw it together and you'll be thanking me for hours afterwards.

The use of garlic does allow me to recommend one of the rare kitchen gadgets we bought that we still use at least twice a week: a stainless-steel soap for washing your fingers with after handling garlic to stop them honking. It sits atop our kitchen sink looking for all the world like a discreet sex-toy, and we love it. The fact that it removes the garlic smell from my fingers (allowing their natural prawn cocktail stink to shine through) is a wonder that science can probably explain, but I prefer the mystery.

Mind, we are suckers for a crap gadgets: our cupboards are memorials to all sorts of tat. One of my personal favourites, bought on one of my customary whims, is our egg cuber. You boil an egg, pop it inside this device, tighten the sides and out pops a square egg. If you think of the number of times you've longed for a square egg in your dinner, it's worth almost any price.

It says a lot about some of the folks in our group that we got away with saying square eggs were an actual brand you could buy in Waitrose, though. Imagine being a poor hen having to plop that out!

4 tbsp honey
4 tbsp beef stock
1 tbsp mirin
1 tbsp light or dark soy sauce
500g (1lb 2oz) stir-fry beef strips
5 cloves of garlic, finely chopped
½ tsp dried chilli flakes

In a bowl, mix together the honey, beef stock, mirin and soy sauce, and set aside.

Spray a large frying pan with a little oil and place it over a medium heat. Add the beef and cook for 2–3 minutes, stirring frequently, then remove and set aside.

Add the garlic to the pan and cook for 30 seconds.

Add the sauce mix to the pan and bring to the boil. Simmer for 2–3 minutes, or until it has thickened, then remove from the heat.

Put the beef back into the pan and stir well to coat.

Sprinkle over the chilli flakes and serve.

NOTE

Serve with rice or noodles.

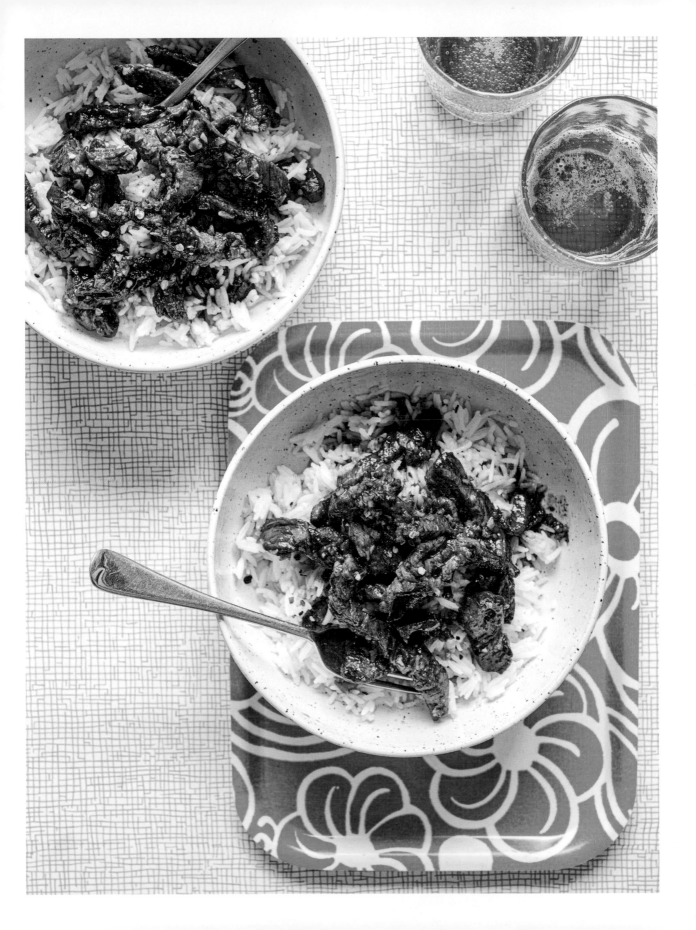

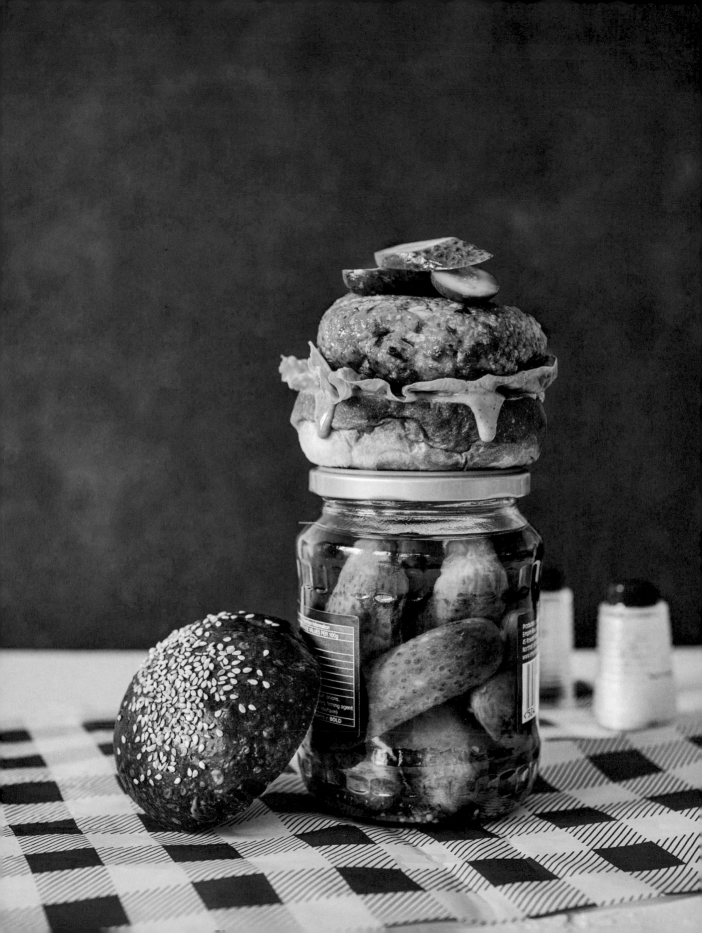

ZESTY SALMON BURGERS

SERVES: 4
PREP: 10 minutes
COOK: 10 minutes
CALORIES: 484

I think everyone has their own unique childhood barbecue experiences. We always had, without fail, a sad little green Tupperware bowl (which had a double life as the vomit bowl) filled with wilted lettuce leaves from the back of the fridge, thick discs of cucumber (flavourless) and quartered, cheap tomatoes that were already wrinkled. Drizzled on top was a magical dressing which was four parts salad cream to one part vinegar (this, actually, is pretty decent and I won't be told otherwise). Alongside that would be a smaller green bowl of 'golden vegetable rice', which was always made far too early in the day so by the time you actually got to it, it would be filled with dimples from falling condensation and hard as a rock. Final flourish? Thick discs of 'French stick', buttered and then covered with a tea towel that had a strong stale-laundry smell to it, so in between picking out fluff from the butter you'd also get a waft of Fresh Meadow. Simpler times.

4 wholemeal buns
1 little gem lettuce, roughly chopped
16 slices of pickled gherkin

For the mayonnaise
3 tbsp extra-light mayonnaise
4 tsp hoisin sauce
4 tsp lemon juice
4 tsp sriracha

For the burgers
400g (14oz) skinless, boneless salmon fillets
50g (1¾oz) panko breadcrumbs
4 spring onions, sliced
4 tsp light or dark soy sauce
zest of 1 lime

Preheat the grill to high.

Mix together all the mayonnaise ingredients and set aside.

Put all the burger ingredients into a food processor and blend until smooth.

Divide the mixture into four and shape into 1.5cm (¾ inch) – thick burgers.

Cook them under the grill for about 4 minutes on each side (toast the buns while you're there if you like).

Split the buns and spread a quarter of the mayonnaise mixture over the bottom half of each of them. Then line each one with the lettuce and top with the burger and gherkin slices as well as the other half of the bun.

NOTE
We usually cook these on the barbecue and they come out beautifully!

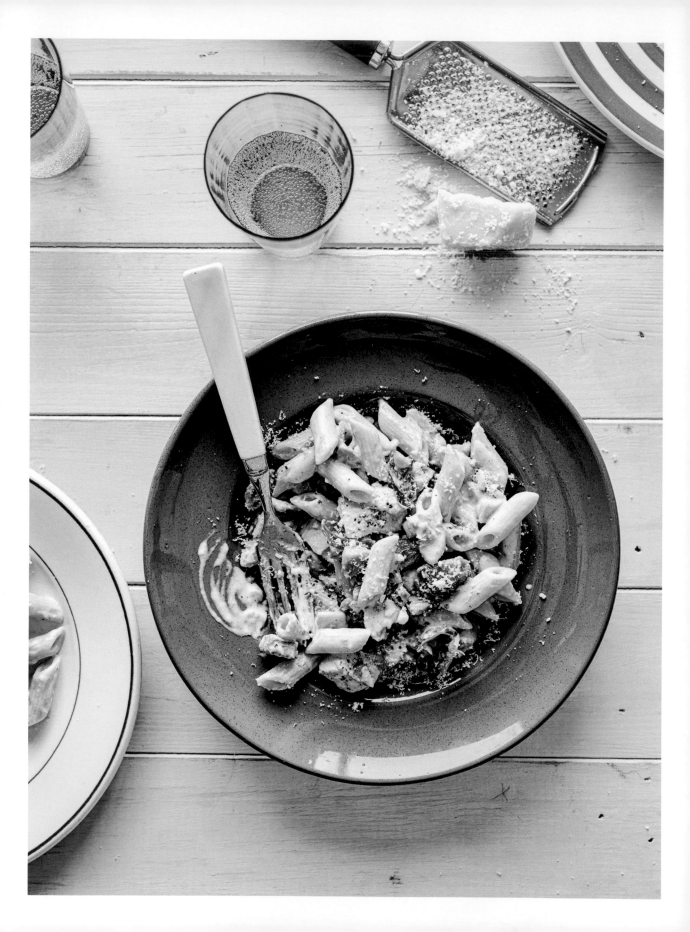

CREAMY QUICK CHICKEN PASTA

SERVES: 4
PREP: 10 minutes
COOK: 20 minutes
CALORIES: 479

A creamy pasta dish is always going to tingle your clopper, and this one, with chunks of bacon and chicken, is a towel-down-job. Doesn't take long to knock this out, though a small note of caution: leftovers are a great idea, but sauces made with cream cheese tend to 'clag' a little the next day. If you're strong-willed enough to even have leftovers, stir a little warm water through as you're reheating.

Leftovers are a nonsense in our house anyway: it doesn't matter if we cook for two or eight, if there's food left we're having it. The four or so hours between our evening meal and going to bed is punctured by the sound of the oven door opening and the two of us snaffling whatever is left, independent of one another. Then, when it comes to portioning up for lunch the next day, we both have to feign ignorance despite knowing the other is as guilty.

The cats usually get the blame.

225g (8oz) pasta
2 skinless, boneless chicken breasts, diced
4 bacon medallions, diced
3 cloves of garlic, crushed
½ chicken stock cube, dissolved in 60ml (2fl oz) hot water
125g (4½oz) extra-light soft cheese
125g (4½oz) cherry tomatoes
3 tbsp Parmesan cheese, grated

Cook the pasta according to the packet instructions, drain and set aside.

Meanwhile, heat a frying pan over a medium-high heat and spray it with a little oil. Add the chicken to the pan and cook for 3–4 minutes, until cooked. Remove from the pan and set aside.

Add the bacon to the pan and fry until cooked.

Add the garlic, cook for 20 seconds, then pour in the chicken stock and simmer for 1 minute.

Add the soft cheese and cherry tomatoes and cook for 3–4 minutes.

Put the chicken back into the pan and cook for a few more minutes.

Stir in the pasta, and sprinkle over the Parmesan.

Serve.

SMART SWAP

Whatever pasta you have stashed in your cupboard will do! Penne and tagliatelle are good shouts.

5 THINGS TO DO WITH YOGHURT

In our continuing theme of '5 things to do with …', we turn now to the humble yoghurt. How often do we find ourselves at the end of a week with a pot of uneaten natural yoghurt peering at us from the fridge? Well, fret no more, wasteful one – we've come up with five simple ideas to use it up.

Just a quick word, though: although we use and champion fat-free yoghurt in our recipes, we have absolutely no guilt picking up the full-fat stuff if we're in a rush. Calorie-wise there's not a massive difference, and fat-free tends to mean they've replaced that delicious fat with sugars and sweeteners. But you do you, love.

MAKES: 10 shards
PREP: 3 hours
COOK: 0 minutes
CALORIES: 40
DIET: VEG

NOTE

Fat-free yoghurt doesn't work as well. Splash out a bit on the good stuff.

YOGHURT BARK

250g (9oz) natural yoghurt
1 tbsp honey
¼ tsp vanilla extract
a handful of sliced strawberries,
    blueberries, raspberries
a small handful of Rice Krispies
    or cornflakes, roughly crushed

Line a baking tray with greaseproof paper.

In a bowl, mix together the yoghurt, honey and vanilla extract, then spread out on the baking sheet to an even thickness.

Sprinkle the berries and cereal on top and freeze for 2–3 hours.

Break into shards and serve.

SERVES: 4
PREP: 5 minutes
COOK: 0 minutes
CALORIES: 29
DIET: VEG/GF

RAITA

125g (4½oz) natural yoghurt
70g (2½oz) cucumber, deseeded and
    diced
½ spring onion, finely chopped
¼ tsp ground coriander
¼ tsp ground cumin
1 tbsp chopped fresh coriander leaves

Mix everything together in a bowl, then chill until needed.

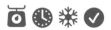

MANGO LASSI

200g (7oz) natural yoghurt
100ml (3½fl oz) milk
150g (5½oz) diced mango
2 tsp honey
a handful of ice (optional)

Put all the ingredients into a blender and blend for 1–2 minutes.

NOTES

This is perfect as a side for any Indian dish, or as a snack with some toasted pitta breads.

Parmesan cheese contains animal rennet so if you're vegetarian, use vegetarian Italian hard cheese instead.

SPINACH DIP

600g (1lb 5oz) frozen chopped spinach
500g (1lb 2oz) fat-free Greek yoghurt
4 spring onions, finely sliced
½ vegetable stock cube
40g (1½oz) Parmesan cheese, grated
a couple of grinds of black pepper

Put the spinach into a colander and rinse with warm water until thawed.

Squeeze the ever-living hell out of the spinach. If you think you've finished, squeeze again.

Once suitably squeezed, stir it into the yoghurt and add the spring onions, crumbled stock cube, Parmesan cheese and black pepper.

Mix well and serve.

NOTE

Use absolutely anything you like – we particularly love blueberries or banana with vanilla yoghurt, or raspberries and blackberries with coconut yoghurt.

LOLLIES

500g (1lb 2oz) fat-free Greek yoghurt
1 tbsp honey
a handful of blueberries (see note)

Mix the ingredients together, pour into moulds, and freeze for at least 2 hours or until solid.

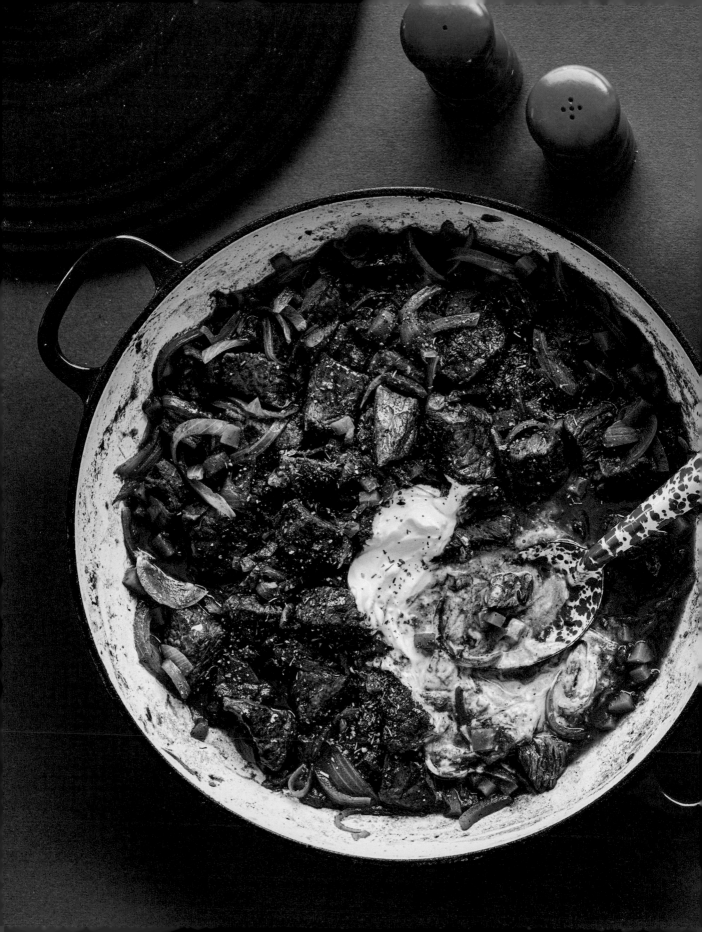

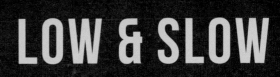

LOW & SLOW

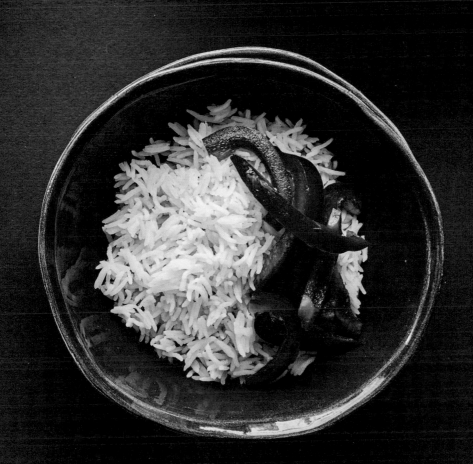

JAMAICAN JERK CHICKEN

SERVES: 4
PREP: 5 minutes
COOK: 30 minutes
CALORIES: 471

1 kg (2lb 4oz) skinless,
  boneless chicken thighs
1 tbsp rum
100ml (3½oz) chicken stock
1 lime, quartered

For the rub
3 tbsp onion powder
3 tbsp dried thyme
3 tbsp ground allspice
3 tbsp black pepper
2 tbsp brown sugar
2 tbsp garlic granules
1 tbsp salt
1 tbsp ground ginger
1 tbsp ground cinnamon
1 tbsp grated nutmeg
1½ tbsp cayenne pepper
1 tbsp dried marjoram
1 tbsp dried sage
1 tbsp dried rosemary

We always include a recipe where the ingredients list is as long as my reasons for not sticking to my wedding vows, but as we reference at the start of the book, a well-stocked spice cupboard is never a bad thing.

This recipe is delicious: but if you're stuck for time, a jerk rub from the supermarket will do the job. I'd exercise caution telling folks you're sneaking out to Tesco for a jerk rub, mind you …

Mix together all the rub ingredients and rub into the chicken thighs.

Heat a large ovenproof pan over a high heat and spray it with a little oil. Add the thighs to the pan and cook for 4–5 minutes, then turn them over and cook for another 5 minutes.

Remove the pan from the heat, then pop it into the oven and cook for 15 minutes.

Stir the rum into the stock, pour into the pan and put back into the oven for another 10 minutes.

Remove and allow to rest for 5 minutes. Divide between four plates and squeeze over the wedges of lime.

NOTES

This is a long list of ingredients, granted, but we promise the taste is out of this world. It's worth it!

Serve with rice.

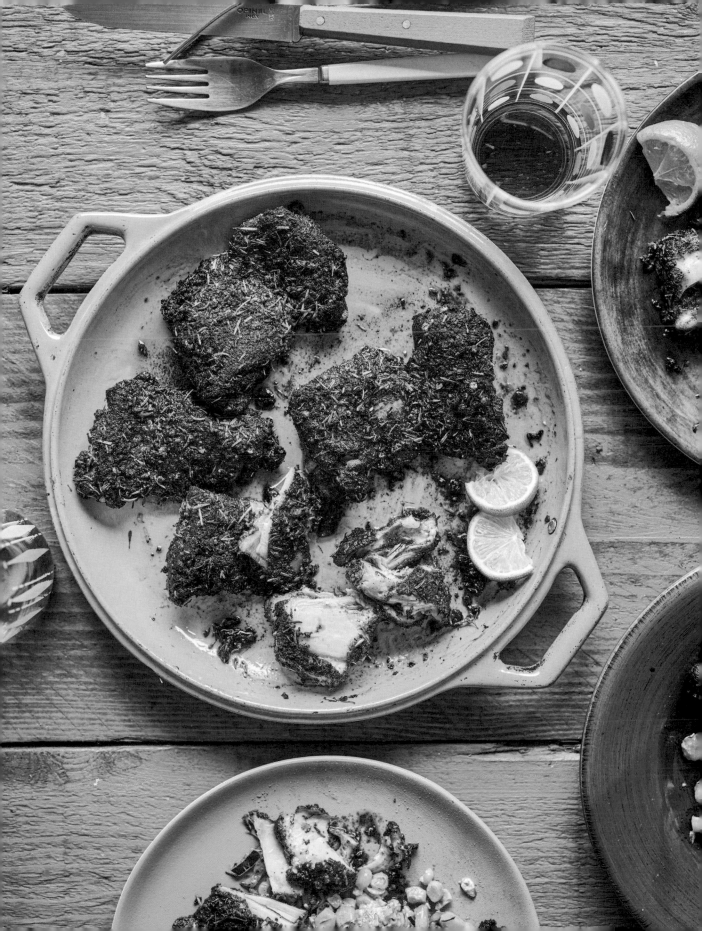

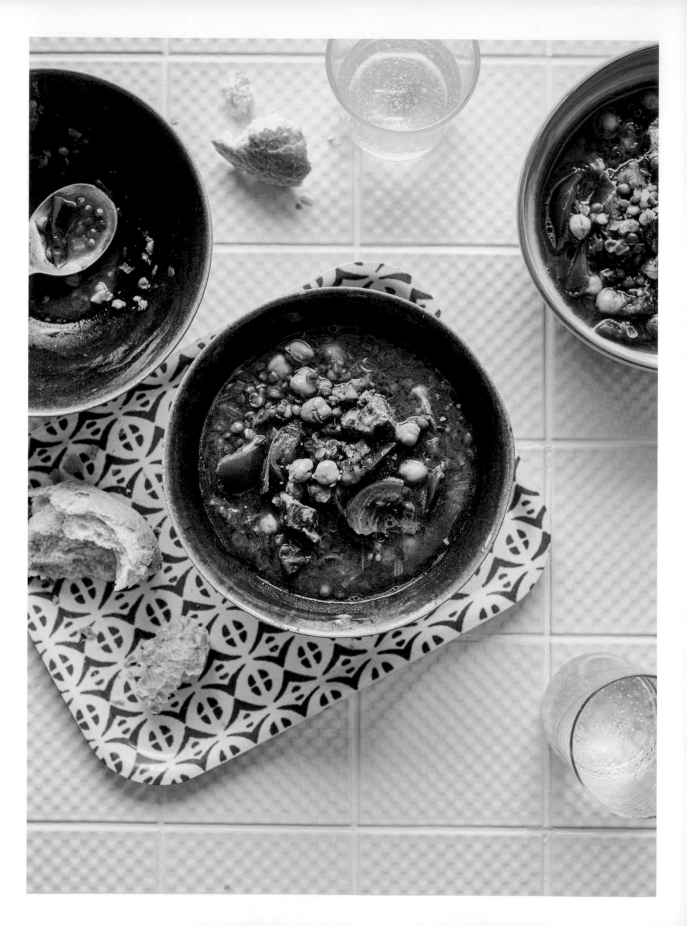

MOROCCAN SOUP

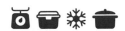

SERVES: 4
PREP: 10 minutes
COOK: 30 minutes
CALORIES: 485

This tasty little soup uses lamb and a pressure cooker, but you can swap it for chicken if you're precious. If you're vegetarian, use butternut squash and vegetable stock cubes instead. The 'meat' isn't the star of the dish here, it's the combination of all the spices that turns this soup into a cup of tagine goodness. If you don't have a pressure cooker, don't sweat it – or rather do – just cook for a good couple of hours in a pan over a bubbling heat.

We first made this the morning before a radio interview and, though tremendous, it does give you heavily-scented little burps afterwards. That in itself would be entirely by the by, but a radio studio is a sealed room and plus, when I'm nervous, I tend to gulp air when I talk. This created the unfortunate sight of the wonderfully professional radio presenter crinkling her nose and visibly blanching every time I loudly exclaimed, which as you can imagine is an awful lot. We were invited back, but use this as a lesson for afterwards: take some Polo mints.

As an aside, I bloody love doing radio: our brief appearances on TV are exercises in trying to make sure Paul's chins aren't avalanching and fretting about keeping my eyes straight. Radio is perfect: we can turn up in our Florence & Fred shirts, barrel out some snappy anecdotes and be sent on our way with whatever props we've managed to half-inch from the studio.

1 onion, finely diced
2.5cm (1 inch) ginger, finely grated
1 tsp ground cumin
¼ tsp grated nutmeg
½ tsp smoked paprika
¼ tsp cayenne pepper
500g (1lb 2oz) diced lamb
150g (5½oz) dried brown lentils
1 × 400g (14oz) tin of chickpeas, drained
4 tomatoes, diced
2 chicken stock cubes, dissolved in 1.5 litres (2½ pints) hot water
1 tbsp cornflour

Select the 'sauté' option on your pressure cooker.

Spray with a little oil, then add the onion and cook for about 5 minutes.

Add the ginger, cumin, nutmeg, paprika and cayenne pepper and stir well. Add the lamb and cook for 10 minutes, stirring frequently.

Add the lentils, chickpeas, tomatoes and stock and stir well.

Cook on high pressure for 15 minutes, then release the pressure.

Dissolve the cornflour in 2 tablespoons of water and stir into the mixture until thickened.

Serve.

SMART SWAP

If you can't find brown lentils, then green will do just fine!

LOW & SLOW

FRUITY FAUX PULLED PORK BURGERS

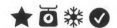

SERVES: 4
PREP: 5 minutes
COOK: 2 hours 15 minutes
CALORIES: 421
DIET: VEG/DF

This is a new take on our famous pulled pork burgers using jackfruit, which seems to be absolutely everywhere at the moment.

Jackfruit is a curious little dickens though: it reminds me of tuna to look at, but pulled apart it really does go 'porky'. Paul is much the same. As a result, using it for these pulled pork burgers wasn't a risk at all – it soaks up flavour so terribly well. That said, if you're someone for whom a day isn't complete without a length of pork inside you, then swap it out for a kilo of pork tenderloin and cook for around eight hours.

2 × 400g (14oz) tins of jackfruit in water, drained and rinsed
1 onion, diced
3 cloves of garlic, crushed
4 tbsp honey
4 tbsp reduced-sugar blackcurrant jam
60g (2¼oz) hoisin sauce
125ml (4fl oz) balsamic vinegar
125ml (4fl oz) vegetable stock
4 sesame-topped buns
4 tbsp coleslaw

Chuck everything (bar the buns and coleslaw) into a slow cooker and cook on low for 2 hours.

When cooked, shred the jackfruit with two forks.

Pour everything into a frying pan and cook over a high heat to reduce it down to a sticky sauce.

Stir, then slop into buns, topped with the coleslaw.

NOTE

You can really serve this fruity pulled faux pulled pork however you want. We've also had this with pasta and it works brilliantly. Be creative!

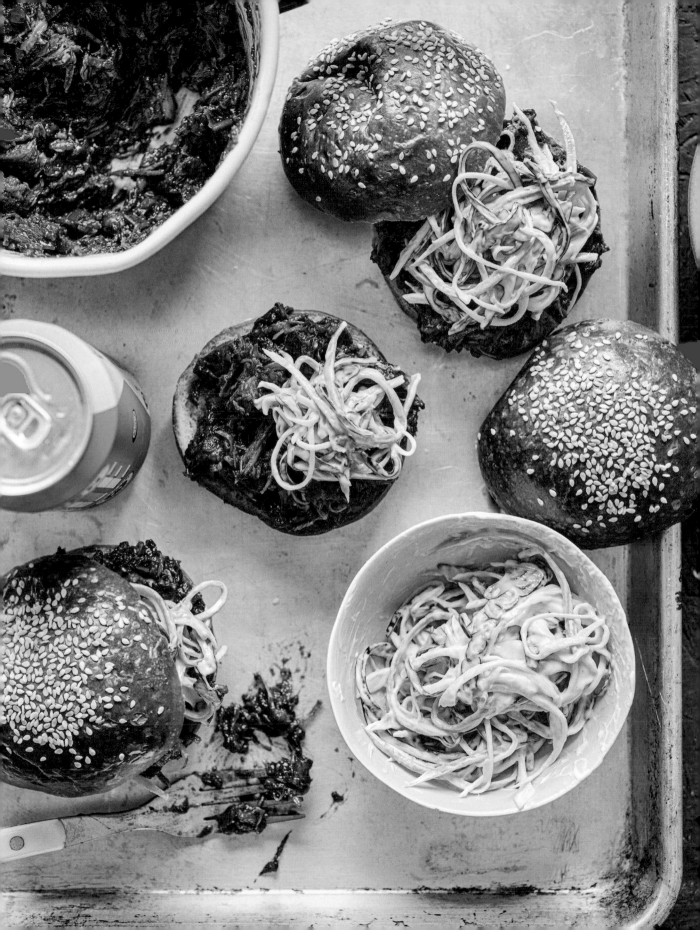

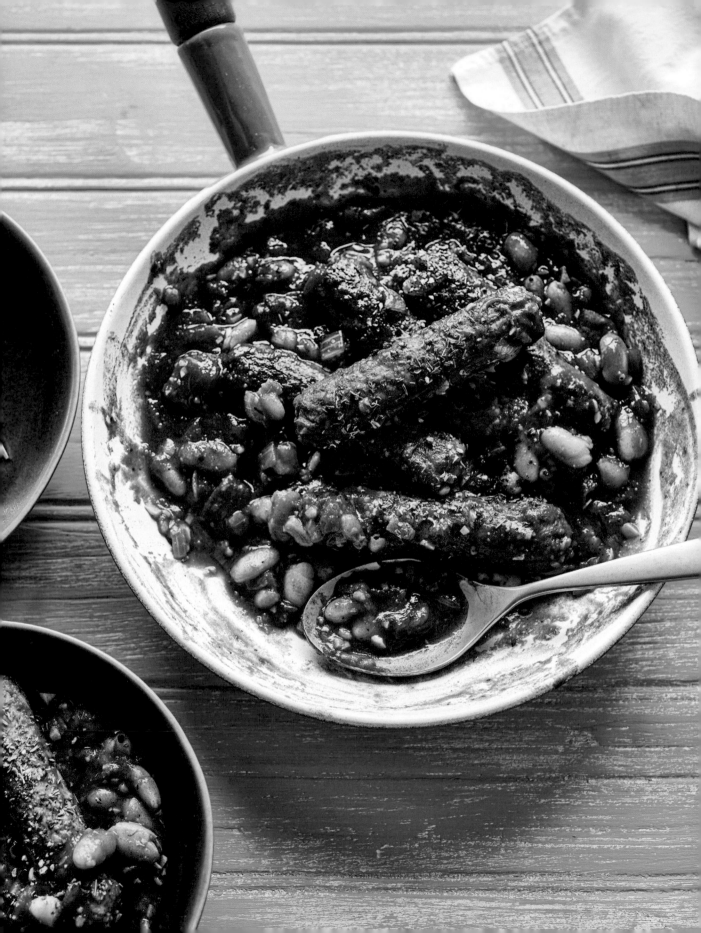

SUPER EASY
SOSIG & BEAN CASSEROLE

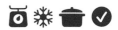

SERVES: 4
PREP: 5 minutes
COOK: 30 minutes
CALORIES: 240
DIET: VEG

Paul insisted on 'sosig' because he thinks he is terribly hilarious. He isn't, but we have to let him win a couple of times.

Paul and I were lucky enough to spend an afternoon making sausages on a nearby farm: it went as well as you'd expect. The Jacinta and Tarquin brigade was taking it all terribly sensibly and making art-gallery frowns in all the right places. We, on the other hand, were shushed and tutted at for being immature and making jokes about willies.

But you know, we are who we are. You put a slimy, loose-skinned tube of meat in our hands and you betcha we're gonna snicker.

Anyway, this is a veggie version of a sausage casserole, because you said the last cookbook needed more of veggie variations – don't say we never listen!

1 tsp fennel seeds
1 onion, diced
4 cloves of garlic, crushed
8 decent low-fat vegetarian
   sausages
1 × 400g (14oz) tin of chopped
   tomatoes
1 × 400g (14oz) tin of cannellini
   beans
250ml (9fl oz) vegetable stock
1 tsp dried oregano
1 tsp dried sage

Grind up the fennel seeds as best you can. If you've got a pestle and mortar – great! If not, just crush them with the bottom of a pint glass or whatever you have. They don't need to be pulverized, just crushed up a bit to get the really good flavours out.

Spray a large frying pan with a little oil and place over a medium-high heat, then add the onion.

Fry for 2–3 minutes, stirring occasionally, then add the garlic and cook for a further 2 minutes.

Add the sausages to the pan and cook until browned (about 5 minutes or so) – they don't need to be cooked all the way through. Add the crushed fennel seeds and cook for a few more minutes, stirring often.

Add the tomatoes, cannellini beans (don't drain them!), stock, oregano and sage, bring to the boil, then reduce the heat and simmer for 20 minutes.

Serve.

SMART SWAPS

Meat sausages work really well with this too, if you're that way inclined.

Use any kind of beans you like – butter beans are great for this, as are chickpeas!

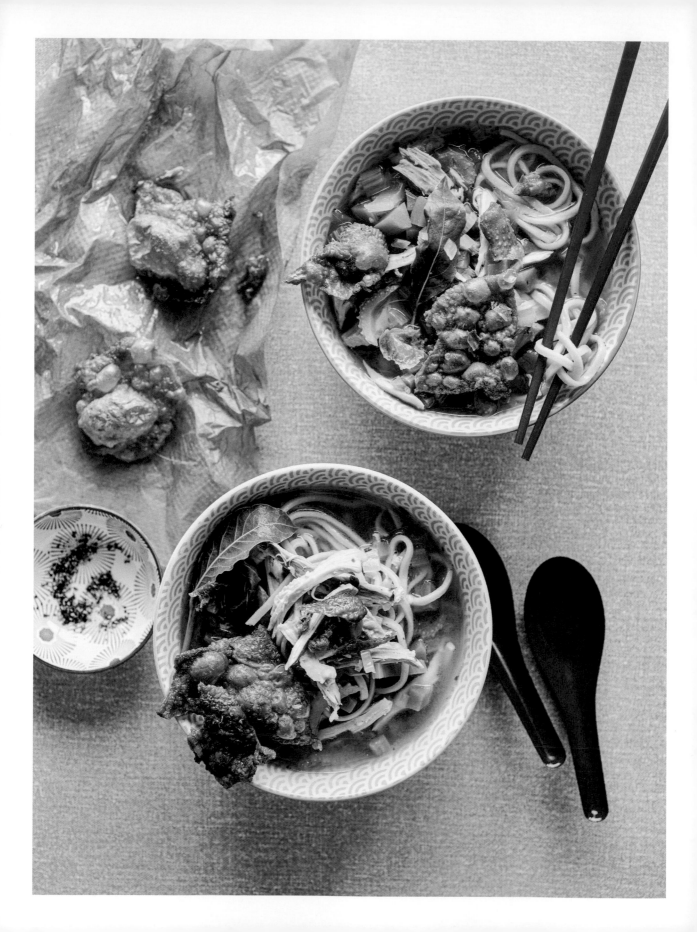

THE BEST-EVER CRISPY CHICKEN NOODLE SOUP

SERVES: 4
PREP: 10 minutes
COOK: 45 minutes
CALORIES: 478

650g (1lb 7oz) skin-on boneless
    chicken thighs
1 onion, diced
120g (4½oz) dried egg noodles
2 carrots, finely diced
4 celery stalks, sliced
3 bay leaves
½ tsp dried thyme
½ tsp dried rosemary
2 litres (3½ pints) chicken stock
1 tsp salt
1 tsp black pepper

Chicken skin splits Chubby Towers straight down the middle, 49/51 – I get the majority vote because I weigh more and I can take Paul in a wrestling match. I'm not a fan, but Paul lives for it. However, it does work terribly well in this soup, especially if you think of it as a particularly crunchy crouton. The beauty here is that the recipe works both ways, so everyone's happy.

If you don't have a pressure cooker, please don't fret: you can simply poach the chicken in the broth as it cooks in a normal pan. Please do make sure that the chicken is cooked through when you shred it, however – we simply shan't be held responsible for any evenings lost to stomach troubles.

Preheat the oven to 180°C fan/400°F/gas mark 6.

Remove the skin from the chicken and lay it out on a non-stick baking sheet.

Try to remove any visible fat from the chicken if you can – this will help with the overall texture later.

Roast the chicken skin in the oven for 30–45 minutes until it's cooked to your liking.

Meanwhile, put the chicken thighs into the bottom of a pressure cooker, followed by all the other ingredients.

Cook on high pressure for 10 minutes, then 'quick release'.

Use a slotted spoon to lift the chicken out of the pressure cooker, then shred it with two forks.

Put the chicken back into the pan, stir well and serve in bowls, topped with the roast chicken skins.

NOTE

If you're not a fan of crispy chicken skin, just leave it out! The rest will still work a treat.

BEEFY TOMATO SOUP

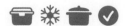

SERVES: 4
PREP: 20 minutes
COOK: 7–8 hours
CALORIES: 323
DIET: DF

We've done ever so many tomato soups (my favourite) in our time – tomato and chilli, ten-vegetable-tomato-soup, tomato and basil – and all our efforts can be found on our blog if you're curious. However, it's not the most substantial of meals, so please find below a more fleshed-out version, which is perfect for the slow cooker. It may not be 'fast', but it takes no time at all to prepare and the reward at the end is worth it.

If you can spare some time, extracting most of the beef chunks at the end of cooking and pulling them apart will stretch the beef still further, but we rather like the chunkiness of the soup as it is. Similarly, a quick whizz around the bowl with a stick blender will smooth the soup out nicely. Up to you.

500g (1lb 2oz) diced beef
1 × 400g (14oz) tin of peeled
    plum tomatoes
5 tbsp tomato purée
1 onion, chopped
2 carrots, sliced
2 celery stalks, sliced
75g (2¾oz) frozen peas
250g (9oz) new potatoes, larger
    ones halved
250ml (9fl oz) beef stock
1 tbsp Worcestershire sauce
1 tsp garlic granules
½ tsp dried thyme
½ tsp dried rosemary
½ tsp salt
¼ tsp black pepper

Put everything into your slow cooker and cook on low for 7–8 hours.

NOTES

You can also make this in a pressure cooker! Brown the meat using the 'sauté' option, then add everything else and cook on the 'meat/stew' setting for 35 minutes.

Alternatively, simmer everything in a big pan on the hob for 2–3 hours.

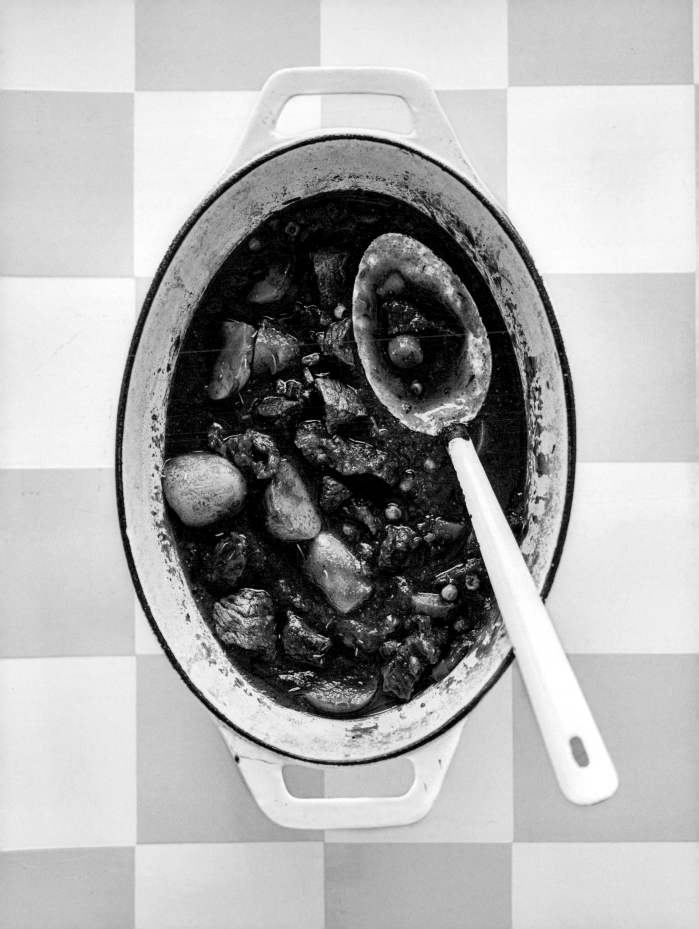

CRISPY DUCK WRAPS

SERVES: 4
PREP: 10 minutes
COOK: 4 hours 30 minutes
CALORIES: 495
DIET: DF

Duck, rather like lamb, is one of those unfairly maligned meats that people cry 'it can't possibly be used on a diet'. Don't get me wrong: I wouldn't recommend ploughing through several at a time like a pig at a trough, but as an occasional treat, it really isn't too bad. If you're trying to reduce the calories, cook it as below so the fat can drip into a tray beneath rather than cooking it on a baking sheet. Every little helps.

We use wholewheat wraps here, but if you can get hold of those Chinese-style pancakes (and most supermarkets sell them), that's far more authentic. Although Paul has eschewed my suggestion for the recipe, I'll give you my own little top tip: once the duck is shredded, I like to absolutely drown it in black pepper. Of course, that's up to you. All I'm saying is: I know my way around shredded duck because I order it all the bloody time in restaurants, whereas Paul once drank the little bowl of lemon water they give you to clean your fingers. Your choice.

1 oven-ready duck, around 1.5kg (3lb 5oz)
7 tbsp hoisin sauce
4 wholemeal wraps
3 spring onions, sliced lengthways
½ cucumber, deseeded and sliced lengthways

Preheat the oven to 170°C fan/375°F/gas mark 5.

Place the duck on a rack or slotted tray in a deep roasting tin and roast for 4 hours. Then increase the oven temperature to 220°C fan/475°F/gas mark 9 and cook for another 30 minutes.

Remove the duck from the oven and leave to cool a little, then shred with two forks.

Spread the hoisin sauce over each of the wraps, and divide the spring onions and cucumber between them.

Top with a couple of forkfuls of shredded duck, wrap and eat!

NOTES

OK, this might not be all that quick to cook – however, once you have done it, you've got a load of duck meat that is perfect for all sorts of meals! We love to stuff it into a wrap because it takes only a few minutes, but it also goes well in our chow mein recipe (see page 178), and loads of other stuff!

You can also cook this at 170°C fan/375°F/gas mark 5 for 5 hours, to do away with the last 30 minutes of extra heat. This is great if you're going out of the house, as you can have it cooking while you're out.

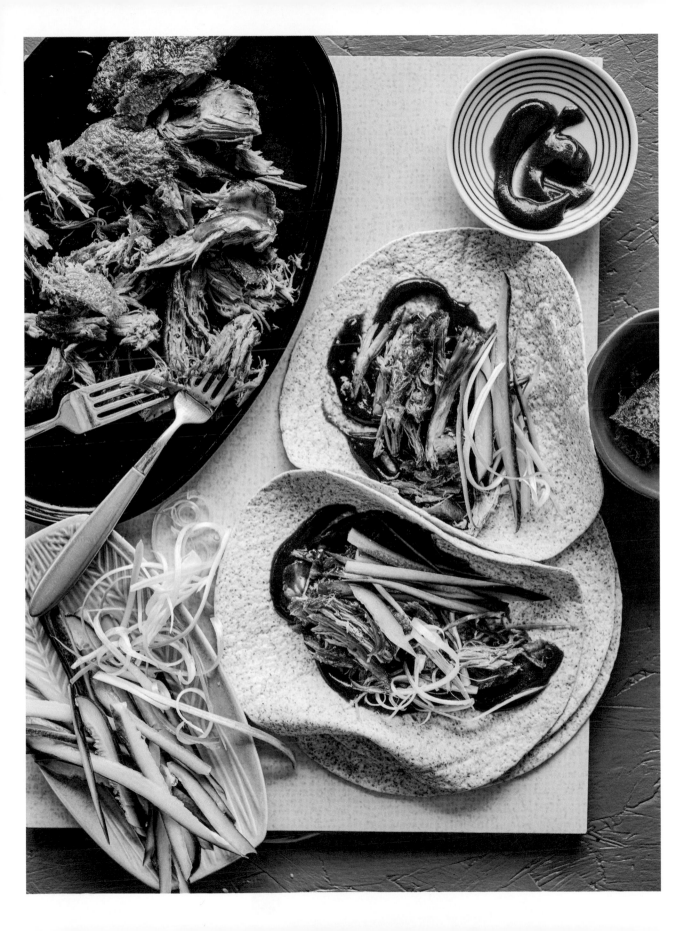

FULL HARVEST SHEPHERD'S PIE

SERVES: 8
PREP: 15 minutes
COOK: 1 hour
CALORIES: 496

Now, let me say something straight off: since we use beef mince in this recipe rather than lamb, this should technically be called a cottage pie. But see, the main twist of this recipe is the sheer amount of vegetables we're sneaking in (hence the harvest), and so the shepherd is staying, damn it.

This recipe is one that has grown over the years in our house. Paul always used to twist his pallid little face that he didn't like vegetables, so like a caring mother with a fussy child, I used to sneak vegetables into meals wherever I could. The tricolour mash is an indulgence that you can easily forgo if you're pushed for time, but I confess it really makes me smile when I see it completed.

This makes enough for 8 large servings, so enjoy some for your evening meal and freeze the rest so you have meals ready to go!

WHAT TO DO WITH LEFTOVER MASH

If you have leftover mash, don't fret, there's myriad of different uses for it:

★ Mash a tin of beans into it and fry off in little patties to serve with brown sauce.

★ Add cheese and onion and bake in the oven.

★ Add shredded cabbage and spring onion, top with mature Cheddar cheese, then bake in the oven for a cheesy colcannon.

Equally, if you have leftover mince, you can turn it into a chilli by tipping some black beans, chilli powder and hot sauce into it and leaving it to simmer.

Of course, the obvious thing to do with any leftovers from this recipe is to make tiny versions of the pie and freeze them individually so you always have a 'ready meal' to hand. But, you do you.

1 large head of broccoli, cut into chunky florets

1 large turnip, peeled and cut into small chunks

4 large carrots, peeled, one finely diced and the others sliced into thick discs

1.5kg (3lb 5oz) potatoes, peeled and chopped into thumb-sized chunks

2 large white onions, finely diced

2 cloves of garlic, crushed

1.25kg (2lb 12oz) lean beef mince

salt and black pepper

1 × 400g (14oz) tin of chopped tomatoes

450ml (16fl oz) beef stock, either from a cube or those fancy sachets from the supermarket

1 × 400g (14oz) tin of butter beans

1 × 300g (10½oz) tin of marrowfat peas

Worcestershire sauce

100g (3½oz) low-fat Cheddar cheese, grated

Preheat the oven to 180°C fan/400°F/gas mark 6.

Set three pans of water to boil – one for your broccoli, one for your turnip chunks and sliced carrots, and one for your potatoes.

The broccoli should only take around 10 minutes, depending on the size of the florets – you want them softer than you would normally have them, as you'll be mashing them.

The turnips, carrots and potatoes should take around 20 minutes – keep an eye on them. Once done, drain and set aside.

Meanwhile, in another large pan, gently fry the onions until golden, then add the garlic and cook for 1 minute more. Add your mince, plus a good pinch of salt and black pepper, and fry over a high heat until cooked through.

Add the finely diced carrot, chopped tomatoes, beef stock, butter beans, peas and a good glug or two of Worcestershire sauce, and allow the whole thing to gurgle and burble away for as long as you can.

Mash your vegetables in their individual pans, then add a quarter of the potato to the broccoli mash and another quarter to the turnip and carrot mash, adding a good twist of pepper to each.

If you want to do this properly, tip the mashes into icing bags with a wide star-shaped nozzle each (or do one at a time).

Tip all the mince into the biggest ovenproof dish you have (you might need to use two).

Top the mince with alternating stars of green, white and orange mash. If you haven't got the time, inclination or patience to do stars, just dollop on pats of each mash and press a fork into them so you get a criss-crossy pattern.

Top the whole thing with grated cheese and cook in the oven for about 30 minutes, until everything is nicely browned and bubbling.

Serve, saving as much as you can bear to leave for leftovers.

NOTE

To make it meat-free, simply use Quorn mince – doesn't taste half bad. 700–1000g will do the trick.

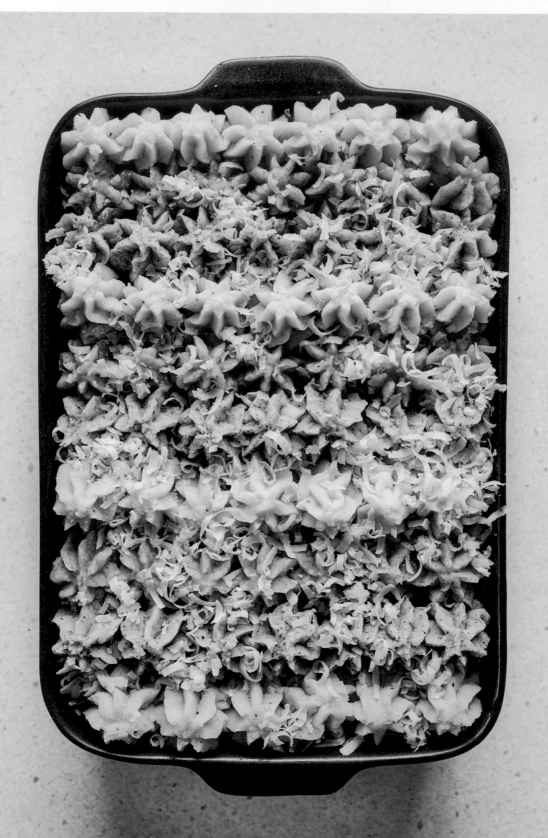

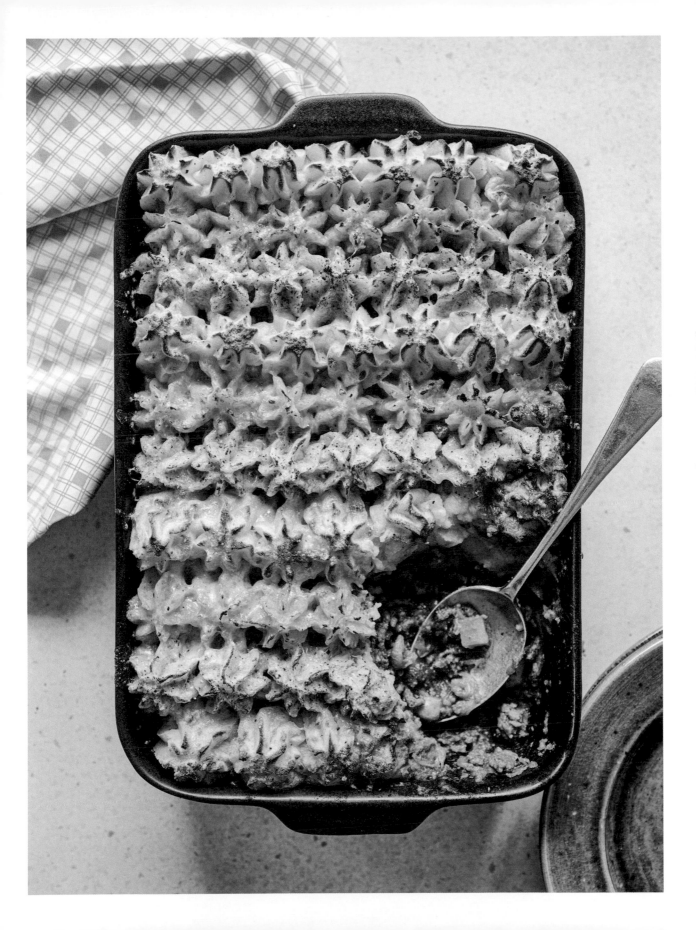

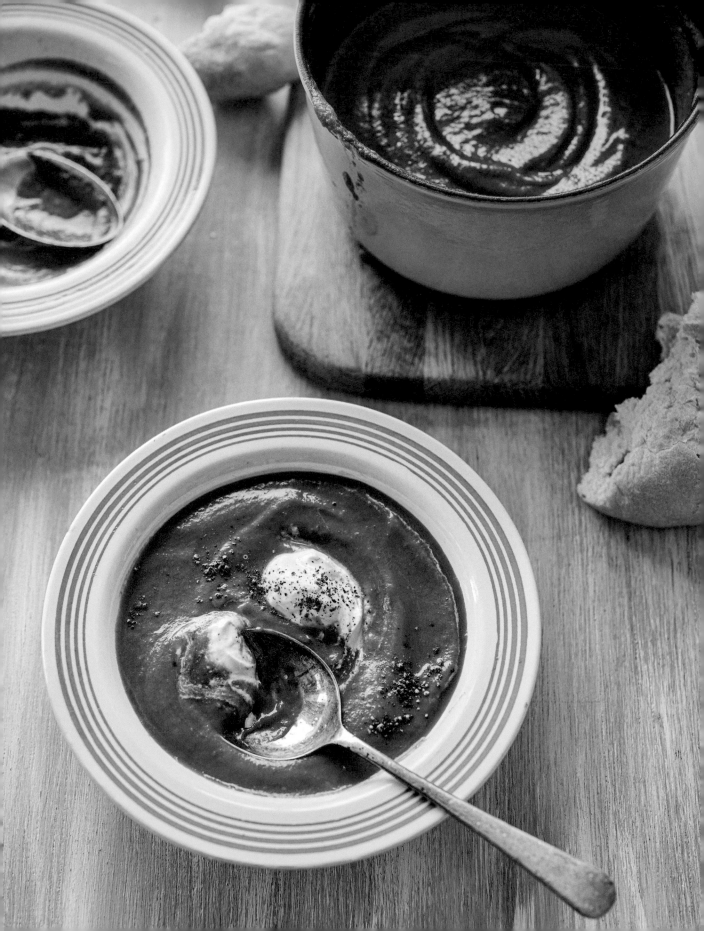

PROPER CREAM OF TOMATO SOUP

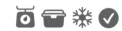

SERVES: 4
PREP: 10 minutes
COOK: 45 minutes
CALORIES: 244
DIET: VEG

This is the sister recipe to the beefy tomato soup on page 90. You may think it's indulgent to have two tomato soup recipes in one book, but while the other is more of a stew, this is closer to the 'famous' tomato soup that everyone knows and loves.

It's terrific because it lets the tomatoes be the star of the show. Please use the best tomatoes you can find: rock hard salad tomatoes from the supermarket that are full of water won't do. Growing them yourself is a doddle if you have a hanging basket, the 'hundreds and thousands' variety provide a feast all summer long.

That said, if you can't get fresh tomatoes, buy the best you can and keep them on the windowsill so the sun can get at them. Tomatoes should never be put in the fridge. It's a paddlin' offence in our house, that.

1kg (2lb 4oz) ripe tomatoes, halved
salt
1 tbsp balsamic vinegar
1 onion, chopped
3 cloves of garlic, grated
1 × 400g (14oz) tin of chopped tomatoes
300ml (10fl oz) vegetable stock
20 fresh basil leaves
4 tbsp double cream

Preheat the oven to 220°C fan/475°F/gas mark 9.

Spread the halved tomatoes on a large baking sheet and sprinkle with a little salt. Drizzle over the balsamic vinegar, along with a good mist or squirt of oil. Roast in the oven for about 25 minutes.

Meanwhile, heat a large pan over a medium-high heat and spray it with a little oil. Add the onion and cook for 6–8 minutes until golden, then add the garlic and cook for 1 more minute.

Add the tinned tomatoes and stock and give it a good stir. Simmer for about 20 minutes.

Next, add the basil leaves and carefully add the roasted tomatoes. Cook for 5–10 minutes.

Either pour the mixture into a blender or use a stick blender and purée until smooth.

Pass through a sieve to remove the seeds and basil leaves, then put back into the pan and simmer for another 2 minutes.

Remove from the heat and serve, swirling 1 tablespoon of cream into each bowl.

NOTE

Look – I can already hear you turning the page when you saw that double cream, but trust us – this really makes it creamy. It's not a lot per portion and it's worth it.

GOULASH

SERVES: 4
PREP: 15 minutes
COOK: 4–8 hours
CALORIES: 454

You can't beat a big bowl of goulash to warm your cockles. I was going to suggest it puts hairs on your chest, but as someone covered almost head-to-toe in body hair, I need no extra.

Take a shower: I can dry myself with a towel for about half an hour, only to put on a T-shirt and discover that my back hair has held on to eight gallons of water, soaking me through. I'm always uncomfortably hot because even in light clothing I'm wearing the equivalent of a mohair jumper. A 'mohair jumper, if you prefer.

I once used three tubes of hair removal cream on my chest and back before attending a fancy dress party as Sabrina the Teenage Witch. Never again – I smelt like a kennel fire for eight weeks after, which was disgusting. I made a cracking Sabrina though, until someone accidentally put a cigarette out on my inflatable boobs (back when I couldn't provide my own). Anyway, to the goulash!

800g (1lb 12oz) diced beef
1½ tsp caraway seeds
150ml (5fl oz) red wine
2 onions, sliced
2 carrots, peeled and diced
1 green pepper, sliced
1 × 400g (14oz) tin of chopped
    tomatoes
4 tbsp tomato purée
2 tbsp sweet paprika
1 tbsp Worcestershire sauce
2 tsp dried mixed herbs
1 beef stock cube, dissolved in
    400ml (14fl oz) boiling water
4 tbsp fat-free yoghurt

Spray a large frying pan with oil and place it over a medium-high heat.

Add the beef to the pan and cook for 1–2 minutes, to sear, then tip it into a slow cooker.

Using the same frying pan, add the caraway seeds and cook for 1 minute. Add the wine, cook for 1–2 minutes, then pour into the slow cooker.

Add everything else (except the yoghurt) to the slow cooker and stir well.

Cook on a low heat for 8 hours (or on a high heat for 4) – removing the lid for the last 30 minutes.

Divide the goulash between four bowls, add a tablespoon of yoghurt to each bowl and serve.

NOTES

If you haven't got a slow cooker or are just a bit impatient, you can cook this in the oven in an oven-proof dish at 180°C fan/400°F/gas mark 6 for 1–2 hours instead.

Serve with rice.

We use the red 'cooking wine' you can get in supermarkets – it adds all the flavour but without any of booze, so it keeps the calories low (and saves the good stuff for later).

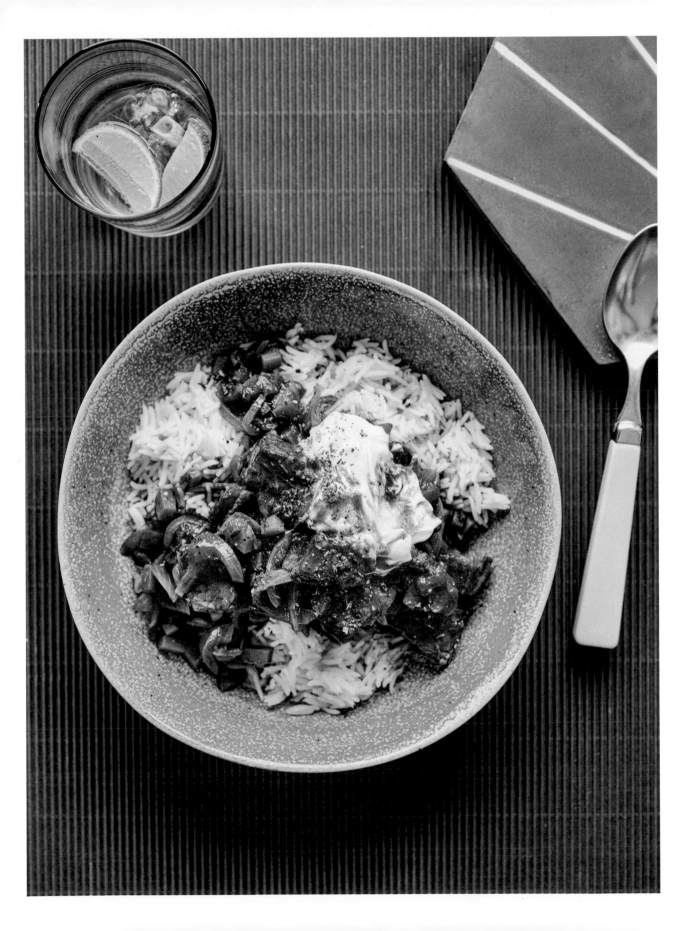

CHICKEN SHAWARMA

SERVES: 4
PREP: 25 minutes
(plus 2 hours marinating)
COOK: 40 minutes
CALORIES: 429

Ready for your family and friends to call you 'big man', 'boss' and 'chief' while they gaze lustfully at your dirty pinny? Cook them this takeaway-style chicken, the idea for which we came up with while carousing around Hamburg one evening. It was 4 a.m. and we were served something similar by the most wonderful man I've ever seen in my life: hands like furry shovels, a neck thicker than both of my thighs combined and a name that sounded like someone extravagantly sneezing into a drainpipe. I fell in love immediately and lit my 'goodbye forever' cigarette with the remnants of my hastily shredded passport, much to Paul's chagrin.

He never called me. To be fair, I didn't give him my number so how could he, but I do hope he sits at the window of Shish Happens even now, tears rolling down his cheek over the memory of what could have been. One day, my love. Meanwhile …

juice of 1 lemon
6 cloves of garlic, crushed
1 tsp salt
2 tsp black pepper
2 tsp ground cumin
1 tsp ground coriander
½ tsp ground turmeric
1 tsp paprika
½ tsp dried chilli flakes
600g (1lb 5oz) skinless, boneless
    chicken thighs
4 tbsp reduced-fat houmous
4 wholemeal wraps
½ cucumber, sliced
4 handfuls of rocket leaves
1 red onion, sliced
30g (1oz) chopped olives
40g (1½oz) feta cheese, crumbled

In a bowl, mix together the lemon juice, garlic, salt, black pepper, cumin, coriander, turmeric, paprika and chilli flakes.

Add the chicken to the bowl and toss well to coat. Cover with clingfilm and pop into the fridge to marinate for 2 hours.

Preheat the oven to 220°C fan/475°F/gas mark 9.

Shake off any excess marinade from the chicken thighs and place on a baking sheet lined with baking paper (throw away the remaining marinade).

Cook the chicken in the oven for 40 minutes, then remove and allow to rest.

Meanwhile, spread 1 tablespoon of houmous over each of the wraps.

Roughly chop the thighs and divide among the four wraps.

Top each one with the cucumber, rocket, red onion, olives and feta, then fold and serve.

NOTE

Don't leave the chicken to marinate for too long – no longer than 12 hours.

SMART SWAP

Add whatever you like to the wraps – we use olives, feta and houmous, but if you're not a fan, just swap them out for your choice!

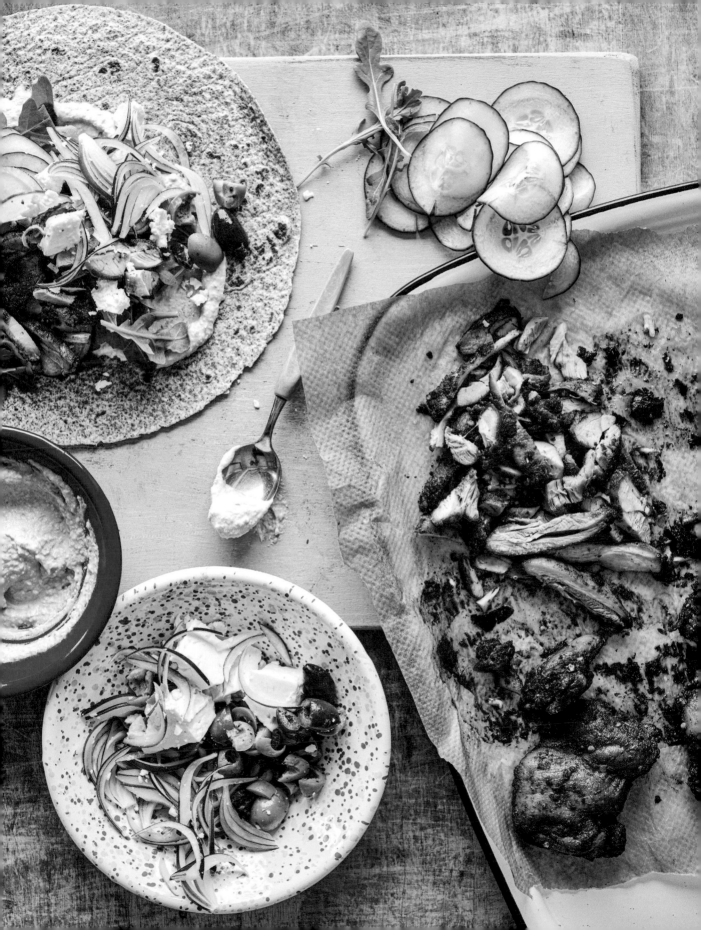

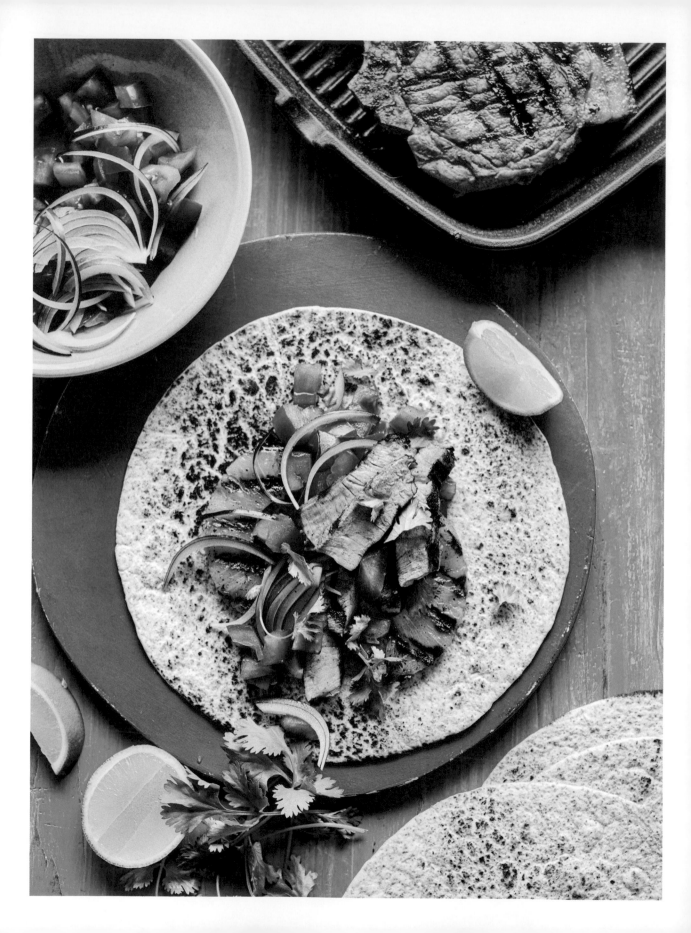

SHEPHERD'S STYLE TACOS

SERVES: 4
PREP: 25 minutes
(plus overnight marinating)
COOK: 20 minutes
CALORIES: 435
DIET: DF

On account of this being a terrifically exciting and complex recipe, I'll keep the intro short, even if it tears my soul apart to do so. These are utterly gorgeous, but it's very much a recipe that benefits from the longest marinade you can afford it. Don't be buying pineapple juice and chunks separately – the juice from the tin will be more than sufficient. This is just as wonderful over rice instead of tacos if you want to drop the calories still further, but we find something comforting about a well-packed taco.

For the marinade

2 cloves of garlic, left whole
2 green chillies, deseeded
   and diced
¼ tsp dried oregano
¼ tsp ground cumin
¼ tsp black pepper
¼ tsp ground coriander
¼ tsp smoked paprika
¼ tsp ground cloves
1 tsp ground turmeric
80ml (2½fl oz) pineapple juice
2 tbsp orange juice
1 tbsp lime juice
2 tbsp cider vinegar

For the tacos

500g (1lb 2oz) pork chops
60g (2¼oz) pineapple chunks
4 wholemeal tortilla wraps
½ red onion, sliced
4 tomatoes, roughly diced
juice of 2 limes
fresh coriander leaves

Spray a large saucepan with a little oil and place it over a medium-high heat. Add the garlic and cook until slightly browned on all sides.

Add the chillies and cook for 3–4 minutes, then add all the herbs and spices and cook for about 1 minute.

Add the fruit juices and the cider vinegar to the pan and bring to the boil. Reduce the heat to a simmer and cook for 3–4 minutes, then remove from the heat and leave to cool for a few more minutes.

Pour the marinade over the pork and leave to marinate overnight.

Spray a large frying pan (a griddle pan is even better) with a little oil and place over a high heat. Add the pineapple and cook for a few minutes, stirring occasionally (it should start to caramelize).

Add the pork and cook for 5–6 minutes on each side (chuck in any leftover marinade too). Remove from the heat and leave to rest for a few minutes, then slice into thin strips.

Warm the tortilla wraps in a pan and top with the pork, pineapple, red onion, tomatoes, lime juice and coriander leaves.

NOTE

To get the best flavour, do marinate the pork overnight – but if you don't have time, you can still make do!

SMART SWAP

To make this one veggie, swap the pork out for jackfruit and it will work an absolute treat.

LASAGNE ENCHILADAS

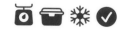

SERVES: 6
PREP: 30 minutes
COOK: 1 hour
CALORIES: 401
DIET: VEG (check mozzarella is vegeterian friendly)

12 lasagne sheets (we use the ones with the frilly edges)
1 onion, finely diced
500g (1lb 2oz) Quorn mince
4 cloves of garlic, crushed
1 tsp salt
½ tsp black pepper
½ tsp dried mixed herbs
1 × 400g (14oz) tin of chopped tomatoes
200ml (7fl oz) passata
250g (9oz) ricotta
100g (3½oz) light soft cheese
1 large egg, beaten
30g (1oz) vegetarian Italian hard cheese, grated
100g (3½oz) mozzarella cheese, grated

Have to keep the intro short for this one because it's a beast of a recipe. I'll share a couple of tips – when it comes to pre-cooking the lasagne sheets, swirl some olive oil into the boiling water if you can spare the calories. It'll stop them sticking together. Another: this recipe uses a lot of cheese, but I don't want you to be scared – you absolutely CAN add even more. Enjoy!

Preheat the oven to 200°C fan/425°F/gas mark 7.

Bring a large pan of salted water to the boil and cook the lasagne sheets according to the packet instructions. Drain, then put the sheets back into the pan and fill it up with cold water to stop the sheets sticking to each other.

Meanwhile, heat a large saucepan over a medium-high heat and spray it with a little oil. Add the onion and cook for 5–6 minutes, stirring frequently.

Add the mince to the pan and cook until browned, then add the garlic, salt, black pepper and mixed herbs and cook for another minute or so. Add the tinned tomatoes and passata, stir, bring to a simmer, then remove from the heat.

Scoop out about a fifth of the mixture, spread it in a layer over the bottom of an ovenproof dish, and set aside.

In a bowl, mix together the ricotta, soft cheese, egg and hard cheese, and set aside.

Drain the lasagne sheets again, and pat them dry with a clean tea towel. Spread them out on a board or work surface.

Divide the cheese mixture between the lasagne sheets and top with a tablespoon of the mince along the middle of each one.

Gently roll up the lasagne sheets (don't worry if it makes a mess) and arrange in the ovenproof dish.

Spread the remaining mince over the top (gently) and sprinkle with the grated mozzarella.

Cover the dish with foil and bake for 40 minutes.

Remove the foil and grill under a medium-high heat for 2–3 minutes to get the enchiladas nicely browned.

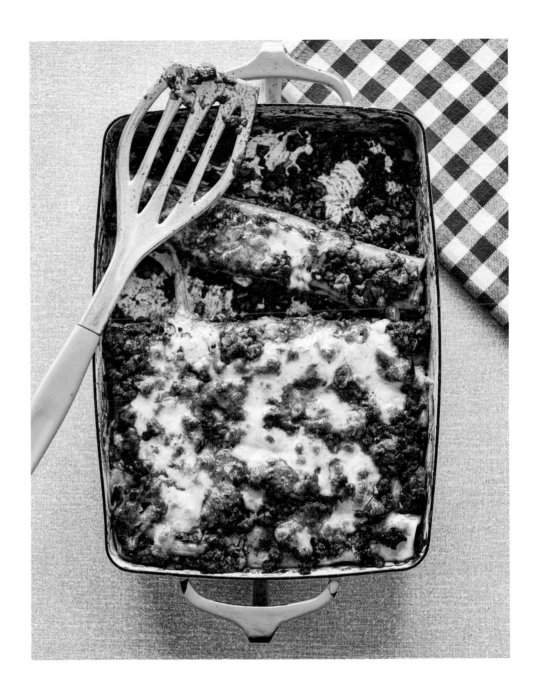

NOTES

We know they're not really enchiladas, don't @ us.

These are brilliant for cooking and dividing up into lunchboxes.

If you want a tasty vegetarian Bolognese sauce, which you can easily scale up, you can make the mince sauce for this recipe and have it with pasta.

SMART SWAP

If you can't get/don't like ricotta, or if you're insane, you can swap out for Quark.

GREEK LEMON DROP SOUP

SERVES: 4
PREP: 10 minutes
COOK: 15 minutes
CALORIES: 354

This lemon drop soup is known as *avgolemono*, which I'm fairly sure I was given a course of antibiotics for back in my wilder days. It's utterly delicious, but a word of caution: it's not the most attractive soup. But reader, if years of living with Paul has taught me anything, it's that beauty is always hidden within. He might have a face like a mine collapse and the warmth of a frostbitten toe, but hot-damn if he isn't gorgeous underneath.

We had this during a fabulous week away in Corsica: we rashly hired a stunning villa in the middle of nowhere (we had just received our mortgage payment and were feeling decadent, what can I say?). The only downside to being in the middle of nowhere was trying to get about in a hire car with all the power and zip of a lawnmower. You've never lived until you've navigated thirty miles of mountain pass in a car that you're almost sure is held together with gaffer tape.

Still, we survived, and this soup was waiting for us in a restaurant at the top of the mountain. It was glorious and now it's yours.

175g (6oz) long-grain rice
3 cloves of garlic, crushed
zest and juice of 1 lemon
750ml (1¼ pints) chicken stock
1 onion, finely diced
250g (9oz) shredded cooked chicken
2 eggs

Cook the rice according to the packet instructions, then drain and set aside.

Place a large saucepan over a medium heat and spray it with a little oil. Add the garlic and lemon zest and cook for 1 minute.

Add the chicken stock, onion and lemon zest and bring to a simmer, then add the chicken and rice.

In a bowl, whisk together the eggs and lemon juice. Gradually whisk in a ladleful of the chicken stock and rice.

Remove the pan from the heat and add the whisked egg mix, stirring well.

Put back over a medium-low heat for a few minutes to warm through, then serve.

NOTES

The trick here is to make sure that it's not too hot – after the initial simmer, make sure it doesn't boil, otherwise the egg will scramble.

You can blend it with a stick blender if you like a smoother texture.

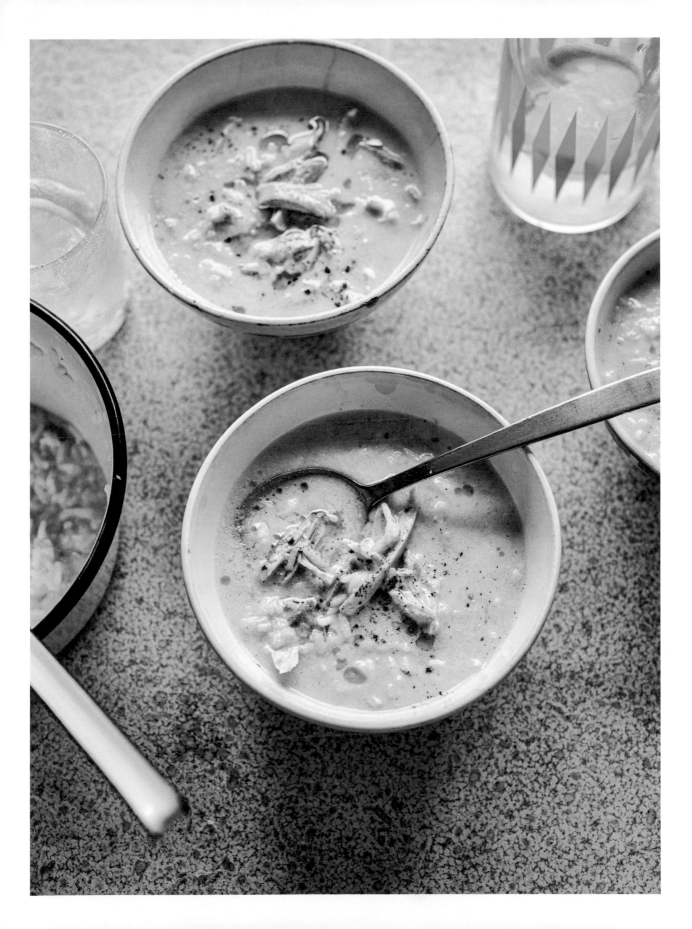

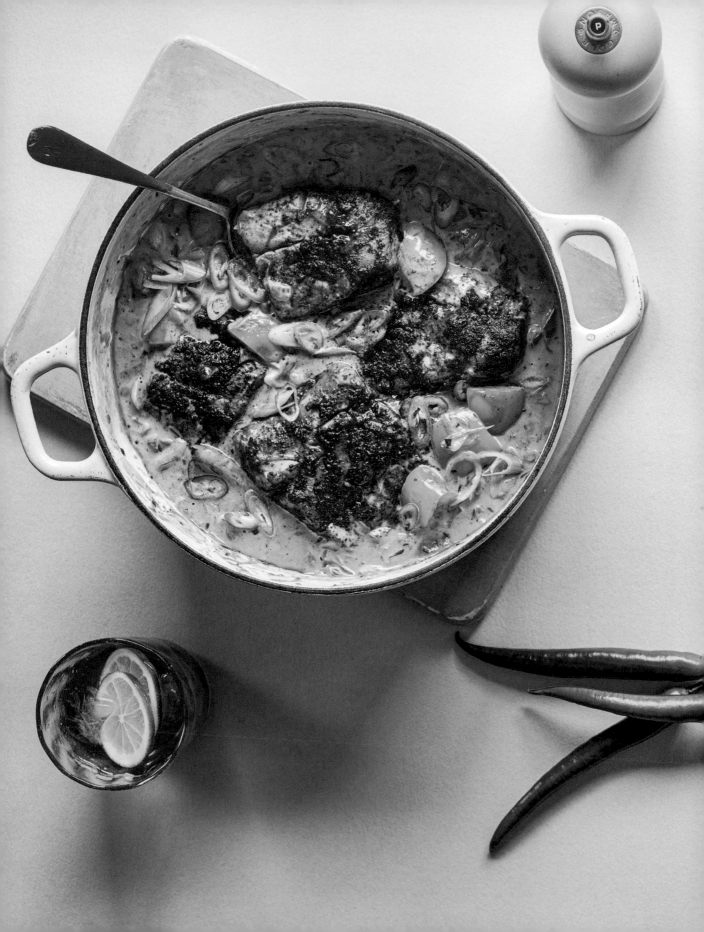

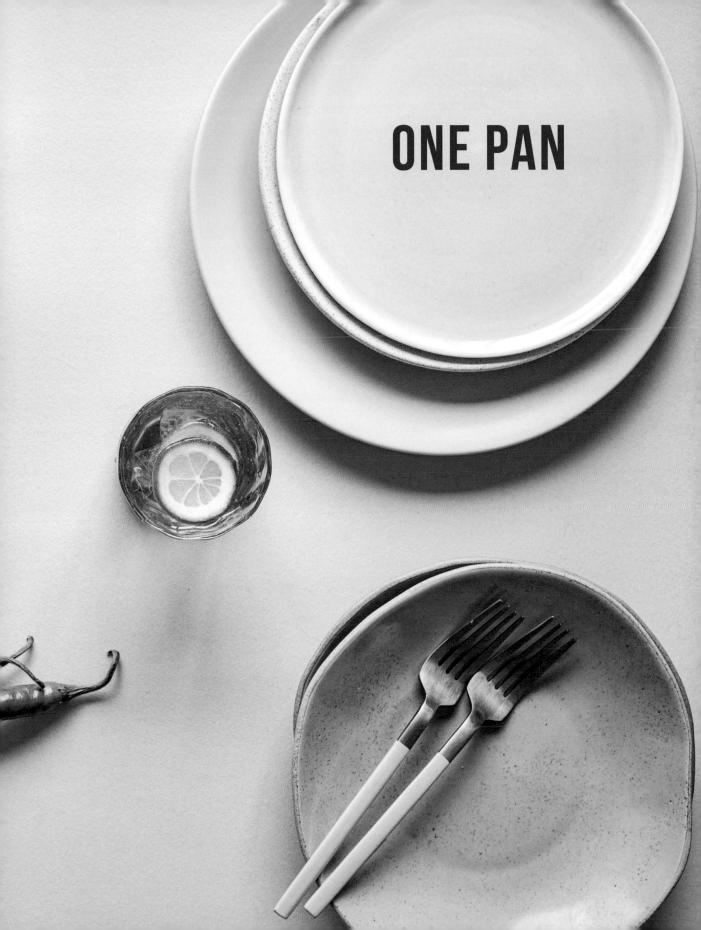

ONE PAN

KOREAN BBQ BOWLS

SERVES: 4
PREP: 10 minutes
(plus 1–2 hours marinating)
COOK: 10 minutes
CALORIES: 282
DIET: DF

Paul made this dish for me the day I passed my driving test, and it's been on firm rotation ever since. If you can get it, pak choi makes a lovely 'meaty' replacement for the spinach, but don't sweat it.

Paul was terribly kind when I passed my driving test on the fifth* attempt. I was all set to pass the first time without incident when I was automatically failed for 'losing control of the car', which was an especially grandiose way for the examiner to note that I'd clipped the kerb pulling back into the test centre. I resisted the urge to lose control of my emotions and bang him out, and what followed was three more eventful tests before I nailed it on my fifth attempt.

Thankfully, all those extra tests have made me a safe, confident soul behind the wheel, a fact I often text Paul about while I'm driving home from the pub. I'm kidding, I promise.

175ml (6fl oz) low-sodium soy
    sauce
4 tbsp mirin
1 tbsp finely grated ginger
1 tbsp sesame oil
1 tbsp honey
2 tsp hot chilli powder
6 cloves of garlic, crushed
500g (1lb 2oz) beef steak, thinly
    sliced
1 red pepper, sliced
1 yellow pepper, sliced
100g (3½oz) spinach
2 spring onions, sliced

In a bowl, mix together the soy sauce, mirin, ginger, sesame oil, honey, chilli powder and garlic.

Put the beef into a bowl and pour over the marinade. Cover with clingfilm and leave in the fridge to marinate for 1–2 hours.

Heat a large frying pan over a high heat and spray it with a little oil.

Reserve 100ml (3½fl oz) of the marinade from the beef and discard the rest. Add the beef to the pan and cook for 2 minutes – don't stir it!

Add the peppers and spinach to the pan and cook for 2–3 minutes.

Add the reserved marinade to the pan and cook for another 2–3 minutes, stirring frequently.

Serve in bowls, topped with the spring onions.

NOTES

You can get away with marinating the meat for 20–30 minutes if you're really pressed for time, but for the best flavour try to get it in the marinade for at least 1–2 hours.

If you're feeling extra fancy, top with some sesame seeds too – it's worth it!

* Paul says sixth time. James says Paul is wrong and will be sleeping in a Travelodge for the foreseeable.

SMART SWAP

Don't have mirin? Rice wine vinegar, rice vinegar or cider vinegar will do.

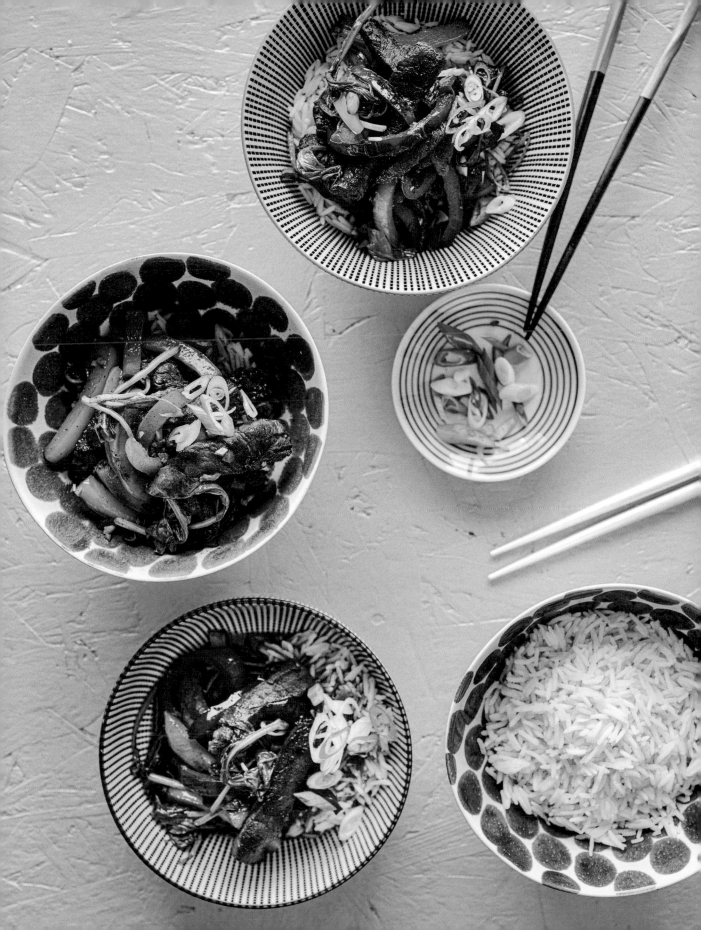

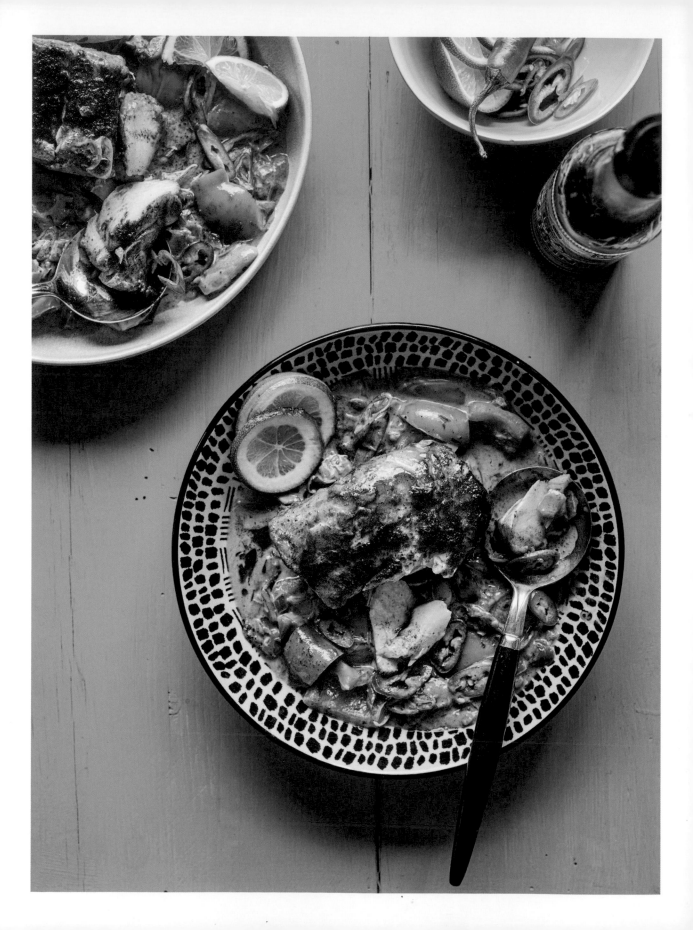

CARIBBEAN COD

SERVES: 4
PREP: 15 minutes
COOK: 45 minutes
CALORIES: 492
DIET: DF

You may have noticed a bit of an uplift in the number of fish recipes in the book: we still aren't massive fans, but you can't deny the health benefits. We've been told for years that 'if it swims, it slims', but Madam, if that were true, twenty years of debauched living would have left us both lollipop-thin.

That's a long list of ingredients, but look – most of it is stuff you'll have kicking around in the cupboards if you're a regular cook. One quick note, because we do get asked this a lot: if you can't find maple syrup, then honey or brown sugar will absolutely do. You may be tempted to swap out the syrup for sweetener, but you mustn't. Happiness comes from within, remember.

1 tbsp hot curry powder
2 tbsp mild curry powder
4 cod fillets, weighing a total of 600g (1lb oz)
2 onions, chopped
4 spring onions, sliced
8 cloves of garlic, crushed
5cm (2 inches) ginger, finely grated
2 yellow peppers, diced
1 tbsp dried tarragon
2 tsp dried thyme
2 tsp black pepper
1 tbsp Worcestershire sauce
2 tsp maple syrup
5 tbsp tomato purée
600ml (1 pint) coconut milk
2 green chillies, sliced

Sprinkle the hot and mild curry powders over the fish and gently toss to combine.

Heat a large pan over a medium-high heat and spray it with a little oil. Add the fish and gently cook for 1–2 minutes, then remove from the pan to a plate and set aside.

Spray the pan with a little more oil, then add the onions, spring onions, garlic and ginger and cook for 5 minutes, stirring occasionally.

Add the chopped peppers and cook for another 5 minutes.

Add the tarragon, thyme, black pepper, Worcestershire sauce and maple syrup to the pan, along with the tomato purée, and stir well.

Add the coconut milk and chillies and give it another good stir.

Bring to the boil, then simmer over a medium-low heat for 20 minutes.

Add the fish to the pan, stir gently and cook for another 10 minutes.

Serve!

NOTE

Dial down the heat by reducing or removing the chilli peppers if you're not a fan.

SMART SWAP

Can't get cod? Any white fish will do! Haddock and pollock are good alternatives.

ONE PAN

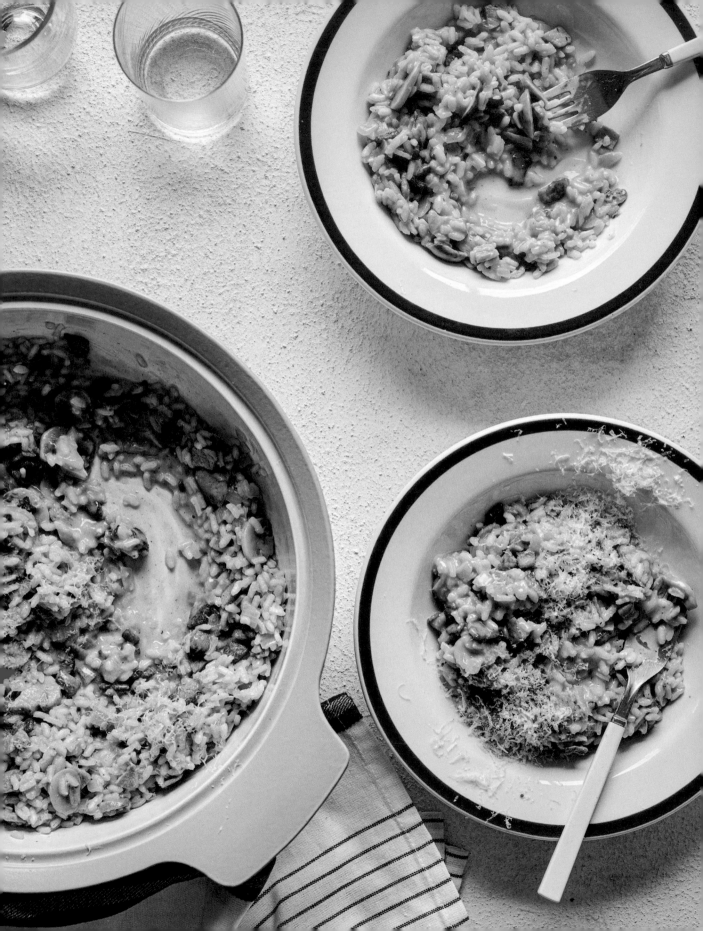

BACON & MUSHROOM RISNOTTO

SERVES: 4
PREP: 10 minutes
COOK: 30 minutes
CALORIES: 498

Long-time readers will be familiar with the concept of our risnotto – risotto but without having to stand by the pan stirring away like a village gossip. I mean, you can do that, but there's really no need – follow our recipe and you'll be rewarded with a creamy plate of pure stodge that'll stick to your ribs.

Not a fan of mushrooms? Nor was Paul, but honestly it's all about finding the right recipe for them. They do look and smell like something that ought to be cast into a fire, but once you get a taste for them, they're grand.

I've always fancied myself as someone who could go into the forest, pluck wild mushrooms and cook with gay abandon (is there any other kind?), but I know my limits. I don't have the patience to studiously examine anything I pick up and make sure it's not deadly: I'd be on the ground thrashing away with foam pouring from my blistered lips in no time at all.

Mind you, I dare say that's how I spend most of my trips to the forests near my home these days anyway, so would anyone notice? To the recipe!

4 bacon medallions, diced
1 large onion, finely diced
2 cloves of garlic, crushed
250g (9oz) button mushrooms, sliced
300g (10½oz) Arborio rice
150ml (5fl oz) white wine
500ml (18fl oz) chicken stock
25g (1oz) Parmesan cheese
3 tbsp light soft cheese
cracked black pepper

Spray a large pan with a little oil and place it over a medium heat.

Add the bacon and fry for 5 minutes, stirring occasionally.

Add the onion and garlic and cook for another 5 minutes, stirring occasionally, then add the mushrooms and cook for a further 5 minutes. Remove from the pan and put to one side.

Add the rice and stir well, then add the white wine and cook for 1 minute.

Add the stock, stir well, then return the mushrooms and bacon to the pan. Cover and cook for about 12 minutes, stirring occasionally, until creamy.

Remove from the heat and stir in the Parmesan and the soft cheese.

Crack over the black pepper and serve.

SMART SWAP

Any mushrooms will do in this, just use whatever you have!

ONE PAN

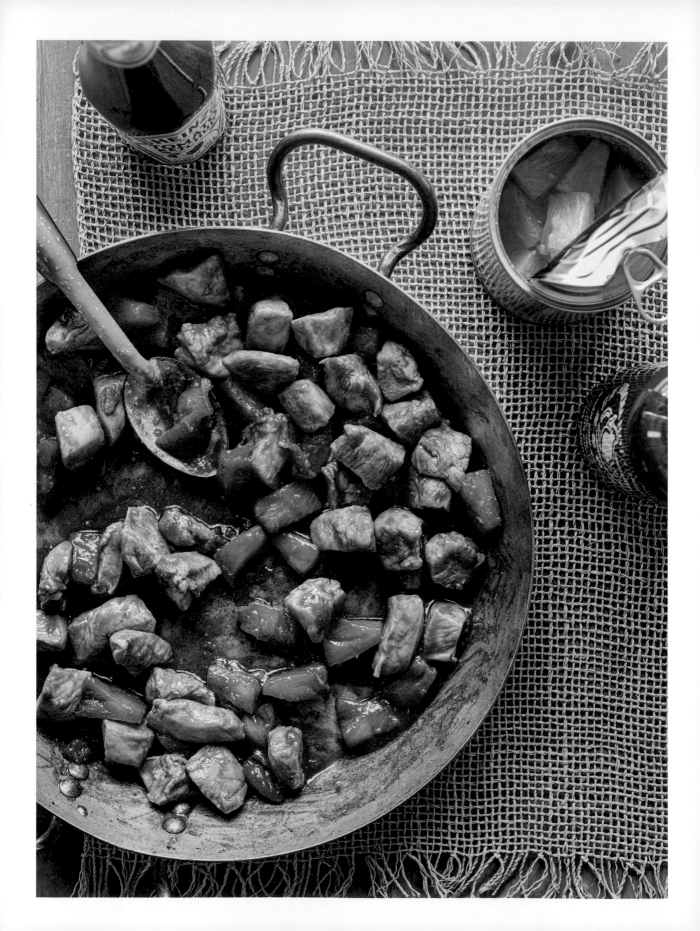

TROPICAL CHICKEN

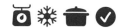

SERVES: 4
PREP: 5 minutes
COOK: 40 minutes
CALORIES: 335
DIET: DF

This recipe was inspired by the stories of a good friend of ours, who spent his honeymoon sailing around tropical islands. He took both his children and wife along (despite me offering to step in so the wife could rest her ankles), and still had a wonderful time.

I nearly got his beautiful, fragrant wife abducted, mind. I gave him strict instructions to return to my arms with bundles of cigars should he happen upon a factory where ladies roll them by hand. To his credit, he found such a place within a day or two, and pulled up his Cadillac outside. Thinking he would be mere moments in the attached shop, he instructed his astoundingly charming wife to sit outside and mind the car.

He was in there the best part of three hours, taking the offered tour of the factory sampling the cigars. The usually placid and understanding Sarah was incredibly displeased to be abandoned, but given she could win a fight with a steam train, there was no real danger. Took two solid days before relations thawed. Look at me though, breaking up marriages from across the world.

Oh, I should say, when he was telling me the story, I asked 'Jamaica?' His reply? 'She didn't really have much choice, I locked the car.'

Cheers, we'll be here all night, try the chicken. Especially the one below.

800g (1lb 12oz) skinless, boneless chicken breasts, diced
200g (7oz) tinned pineapple chunks
4 tbsp pineapple juice (take it from the tin of chunks!)
5 tbsp light or dark soy sauce
2 tbsp honey
2 tbsp tomato ketchup
1 tbsp rice wine vinegar
2.5cm (1 inch) ginger, finely grated
2 tsp sriracha

Spray a large frying pan with a little oil and place over a medium heat. Add the chicken and cook until browned, then remove from the pan and set aside.

Add all the other ingredients and cook for 10–15 minutes, stirring frequently, trying to break down the pineapple as much as you can.

Put the chicken back into the pan and bring to the boil, then reduce the heat and simmer for 20 minutes.

Serve.

NOTE
Serve with rice.

SMART SWAP
Don't have rice wine vinegar? Cider vinegar will do!

ONE PAN

RED HOT TEXAS-STYLE CHILLI!
(AND WE GOT GINGER ALE! BOILIN' HOT TEXAS-STYLE GINGER ALE!)

SERVES: 4
PREP: 30 minutes
COOK: 3 hours 45 minutes
CALORIES: 441

We can't resist a *Simpsons* quote here at Chubby Towers. Barely a day goes by without Paul hollering out a witty bon mot from twenty years ago, though I wish he wouldn't shout them while we make love.

No long-winded intro for this chilli recipe: it's a faster take on our five-alarm chilli from the last book, but the ginger ale adds an entirely different flavour.

A recommendation for moments when you're not on the diet – this, served the day after betwixt two slices of buttered cheap white bread is heaven.

1kg (2lb 4oz) diced beef
1 onion, diced
½ tsp salt
1 tbsp chipotle chilli paste
2 tsp hot chilli powder
1 tbsp ground cumin
2 tsp dried mixed herbs
½ tsp black pepper
4 cloves of garlic, crushed
1 red chilli, finely diced
1 × 400g (14oz) tin of chopped tomatoes
200ml (7fl oz) ginger ale
200ml (7fl oz) beef stock
1 lime

Preheat the oven to 170°C fan/375°F/gas mark 5.

Heat a large ovenproof pan over a medium-high heat and spray it with a little oil.

Add the beef in batches to the pan and brown, this should take about 5–6 minutes for each batch (it doesn't have to be perfectly browned, just make sure it's seared to keep the flavour).

Remove to a bowl while you cook the rest of the beef.

Spray the pan with a bit more oil and add the onion along with the salt.

Cook the onions until they're starting to brown, making sure to scrape the good stuff off the bottom of the pan as you go and mix it in.

Add the chipotle paste, chilli powder, cumin, mixed herbs and black pepper and stir, then cook for a minute or two.

Add the garlic and the diced chilli to the pan and give it another stir.

Add the tomatoes, ginger ale and stock to the pan and give it a good stir, then add the beef, stirring again.

Bring to the boil, stir, then remove from the heat.

Cover the pan with a lid and cook in the oven for 3 hours.

Remove from the oven, squeeze over the juice of the lime and serve.

NOTE
Reduce the spiciness of this by leaving out the diced red chilli.

SMART SWAP
Can't find chipotle paste? Any chilli paste will do, don't be afraid to experiment.

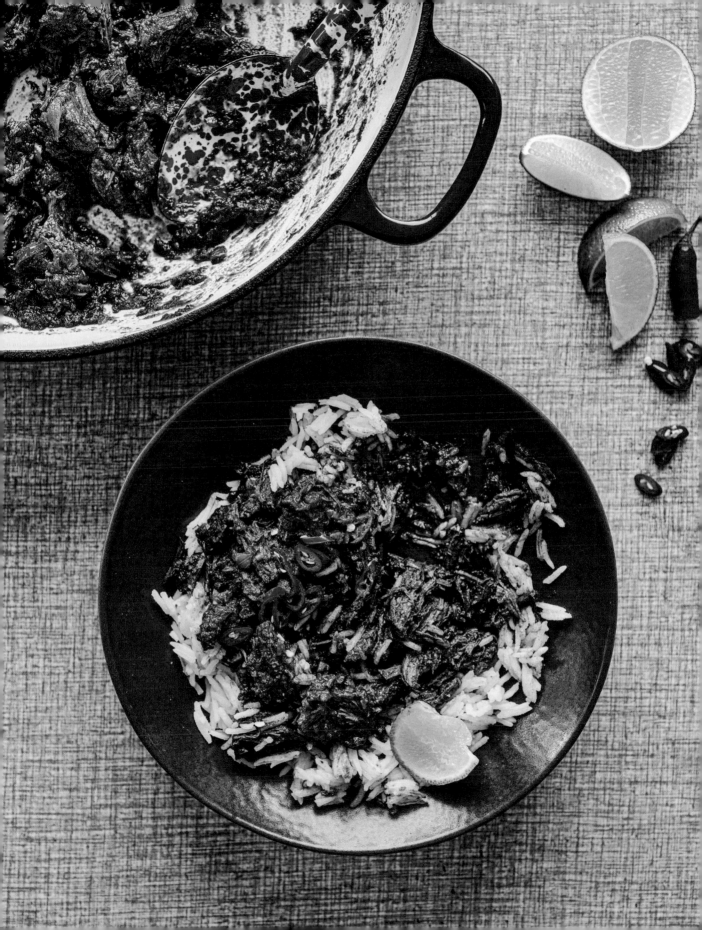

FRENCH ONION CHICKEN

SERVES: 4
PREP: 10 minutes
COOK: 50 minutes
CALORIES: 489

We nearly gave this a fancy title to make it sound more inviting, but damn if we aren't ones for simplistic language at Chubby Towers. French onion soup is a particular favourite of ours, and here we have turned it into a more substantial dish perfect for an evening meal.

Don't get us wrong: there's a time and a place for flowery language, but we both work in professions that lend themselves to saying twenty words when one will suffice and it can certainly make the ears itch. One particular phrase has stuck with the both of us: '*We need that holistic overarching granularity in the round.*'

Forty quid to the person who manages to explain that to us without having a pen poked in their eye. Actually, no: much as I am a fan of targeted workplace acronym tutoring, I think not knowing is even better. You keep it.

1kg (2lb 4oz) brown onions, sliced
1 tbsp balsamic vinegar
1kg (2lb 4oz) skinless, boneless
   chicken breasts
½ tsp dried thyme
½ tsp dried sage
500ml (18fl oz) beef stock
2 tbsp plain flour
80g (2¾oz) reduced-fat Cheddar
   cheese, grated

Preheat the oven to 180°C fan/400°F/gas mark 6.

Spray a large ovenproof pan with a little oil and place it over a medium heat.

Add the onions and cook for 15–20 minutes, until caramelized, then add the balsamic vinegar and cook for another 4–5 minutes (but make sure they don't burn).

Scoop out the onions onto a plate, then place the pan back over the heat and spray it with a bit more oil.

Add the chicken and sprinkle over the thyme and sage. Cook until browned (about 10–15 minutes), turning frequently, then remove the chicken from the pan and set aside.

Pour the stock into the pan and scrape up any bits on the bottom. Reduce the heat to medium-low and gently whisk in the flour until smooth. Cook for another 5 minutes, until thickened.

Return the onions to the pan and stir well to combine.

Top with the chicken breasts and sprinkle over the cheese.

Place the pan in the oven for about 5 minutes, until the cheese has melted and the chicken is cooked.

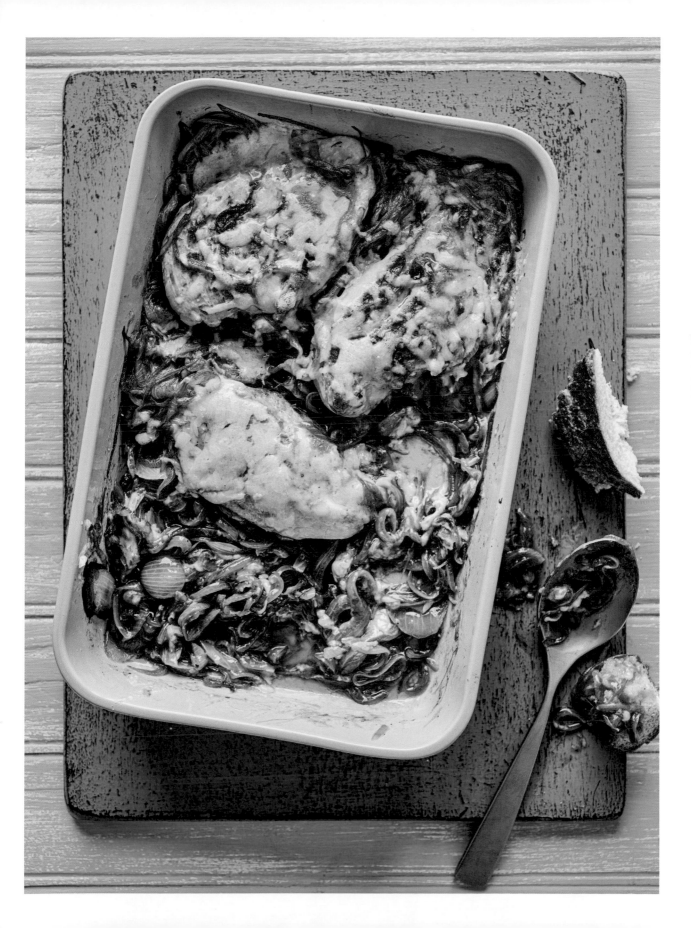

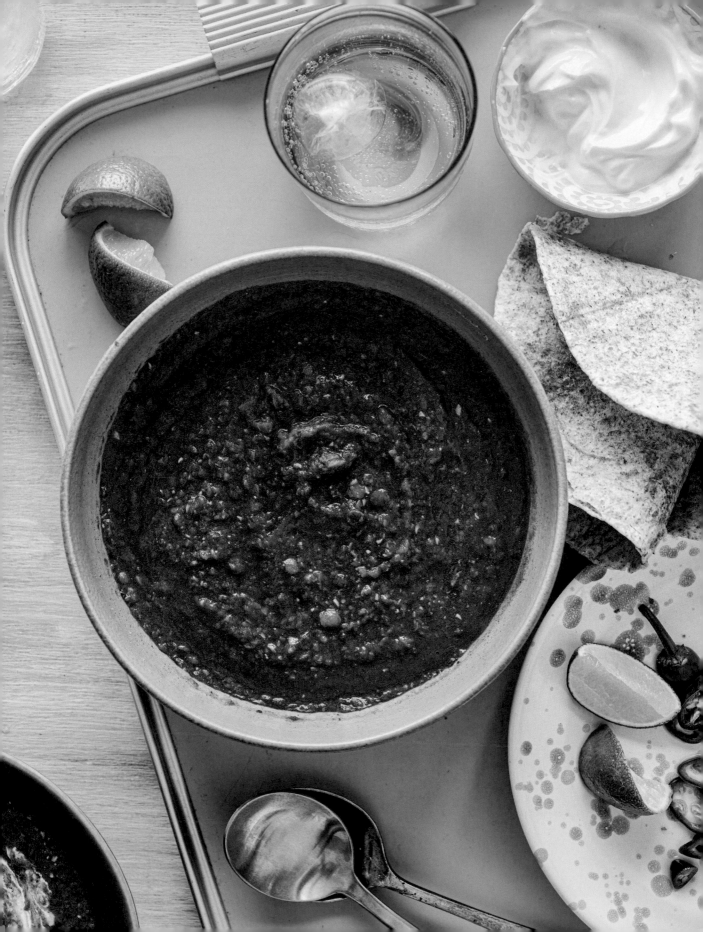

LICKETY SPLIT DHAL

SERVES: 4
PREP: 5 minutes
COOK: 45 minutes
CALORIES: 263
DIET: VEG/V/GF/DF

We've done many a dhal on the blog – there's something reassuring about the ease in which they come together and the fact you can chuck anything in there, which appeals to our hatred of food waste. However, they can be a struggle to 'present', as they look like something that fell out of a sewer overflow.

Thankfully, we have terrific food stylists on hand to make everything look gorgeous, but it raises a wider point that we want to raise. You know when you make a dish and it looks nothing like the recipe? Just remember that recipe books have teams of wonderful souls who will think nothing of spending twenty minutes adjusting slices of chorizo until everything looks just so. Don't be downhearted if your food doesn't 'look as good' – comparison is the thief of joy, and anyway, it all comes out the same!

1 onion, sliced
4 cloves of garlic, crushed
1 tbsp finely grated ginger
1 green chilli, finely chopped
1½ tsp garam masala
½ tsp ground cumin
½ tsp ground coriander
½ tsp salt
1 × 400g (14oz) tin of chopped
   tomatoes
200g (7oz) dried brown lentils
1 × 400g (14oz) tin of kidney
   beans, drained and rinsed
1 bay leaf
1 lime, quartered

Heat a large pan over a medium-high heat and spray it with a little oil.

Add the onion, garlic, ginger and green chilli to the pan and cook until softened, which will take about 5–6 minutes.

Add the garam masala, cumin, coriander and salt and stir, then add the tomatoes and cook for another minute, stirring frequently.

Add the lentils, beans and bay leaf, along with 1.5 litres (2 pints) of water, bring to a simmer, then leave it all to simmer for 35 minutes.

Remove the bay leaf, then scoop out a few ladlefuls of the mixture and blend until smooth. Put the blended mixture back into the pan and give it a good stir.

Serve in bowls, and squeeze over the wedges of lime.

NOTES

For the best flavour, don't deseed the chilli. Get it all in there.

If you don't have a blender you can leave out that part, but it's worth doing if you have one – it makes the texture so much creamier.

This is champion with brown rice, and even a naan or a pitta if you're feeling slutty.

SMART SWAPS

Chuck whatever spices you have into this, don't be shy to experiment!

Can't find brown lentils? Any will do!

Not a fan of spicy food? You can replace the chilli with ½ a green pepper if you prefer.

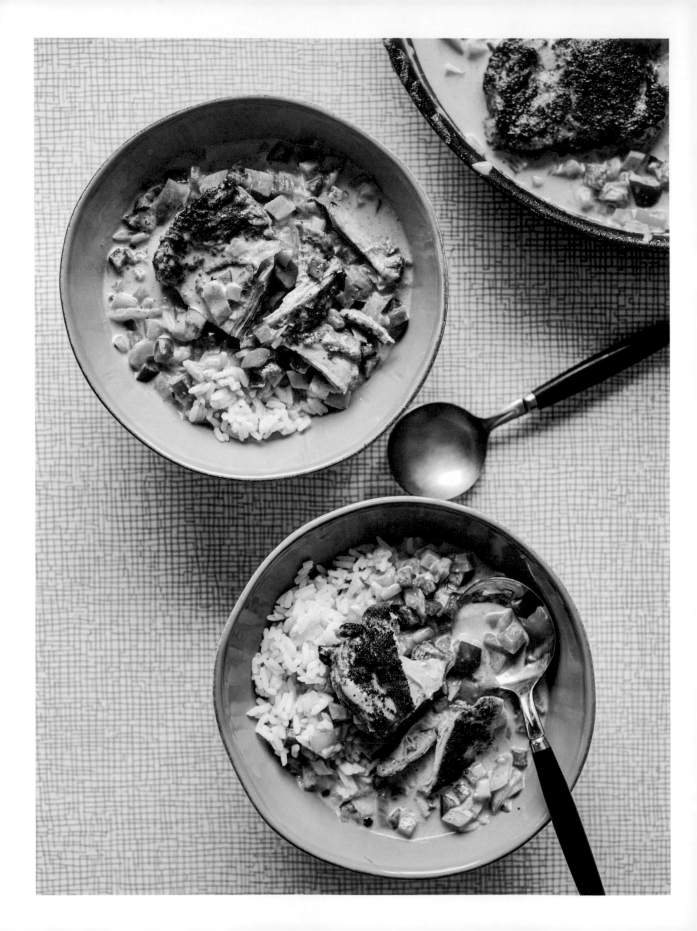

COCONUT CHICKEN

SERVES: 4
PREP: 10 minutes
COOK: 45 minutes
CALORIES: 485
DIET: DF

Gone are the days we would see coconut in a recipe and instantly dismiss it. Coconut milk is high in calories, but it tastes so good that you shouldn't steer clear. We do still leave all the Bounties in a tub of Celebrations, though – who needs that sort of pain in their life?

If you were feeling really decadent, you could buy fresh coconut, though it does seem like a lot of farting on when you can buy a tin. But cracking a coconut is seen as good luck in some cultures, so you could always hope for dieting success as you hurl them around?

I'm not one for superstitions, but I'll tell you a quick little secret: as a kid, I was always terrified that the house would burn down. I watched far too many episodes of 999, what can I say? Anyway, my ritual to ward off the inferno that seemed inevitable thanks to the combination of heavy-smoking parents, an open coal fire and the fact the chip pan was always on the go, was to screw my eyes up before bed, then blink eight times, then clap my hands together six times. Not saying I cracked it, but our house only ever caught fire twice. Not bad …

1 tbsp Cajun seasoning
5 skinless, boneless chicken thighs
1 onion, diced
1 red pepper, finely diced
1 yellow pepper, finely diced
¼ tsp ground coriander
¼ tsp ground cumin
½ tsp ground turmeric
¼ tsp black pepper
2 × 400ml (14fl oz) tins of coconut milk

Rub the Cajun seasoning over the chicken thighs.

Spray a large frying pan with a little oil and place over a medium-high heat. Add the chicken thighs and cook for 5–6 minutes, then turn them and cook for another 6–7 minutes.

Remove the thighs from the pan and set aside. Spray the pan with a bit more oil and add the onion, peppers, coriander, cumin, turmeric and black pepper. Cook for 5 minutes, stirring frequently.

Add the coconut milk, stir, then simmer for 20 minutes.

Put the chicken back into the pan and cook for 2 more minutes.

Serve!

NOTES

Don't be tempted to swap the coconut milk for the light stuff – it won't taste anywhere near as nice.

This is tasty served with rice or pasta.

SMART SWAP

You'll find Cajun seasoning in supermarkets. Can't get it? Any spice mix will do!

STICKY CHICKY THIGHS

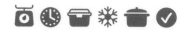

SERVES: 4
PREP: 5 minutes
COOK: 20 minutes
CALORIES: 259
DIET: GF/DF

We talked at length about chicken thighs in the last book, so we shan't bore you again except to remind you that the best taste comes from the dark meat. Breasts are fine, but if you want real flavour, you know where to go.

I'm using this honey-based recipe to make a plea to you all: help save the bees! For years we kept a 'tidy' garden, lawns clipped right back and very few flowers. We hadn't quite gone to the level of some of our neighbours who cut their lawns with kitchen scissors, thank heavens, but it was all so sterile.

Two years ago we decided to ditch that because, frankly, who has the time or inclination to fart about in the garden? Not us, and we have a gardener. So we let it quite literally go to seed, threw a few 'bee bombs' around, which exploded into patches of wildflower, and honestly, it looks amazing.

We have so much wildlife now – not just bees, but hedgehogs in the long grass, butterflies in the shrubbery and so many birds nesting in the trees that are threatening to knock our roof off. It's genuinely glorious, and if I make only one demand of you in exchange for this fabulous recipe book, it is that you give this a go yourself.

3 tbsp Dijon mustard
3 tbsp honey
½ tsp garlic granules
8 skinless, boneless chicken
   thighs

Preheat the oven to 220°C fan/475°F/gas mark 9.

In a large bowl, mix together the mustard, honey and garlic granules.

Add the chicken and toss well to coat.

Place the chicken on a baking sheet and bake for 20 minutes.

Serve.

NOTE
Serve with a side salad.

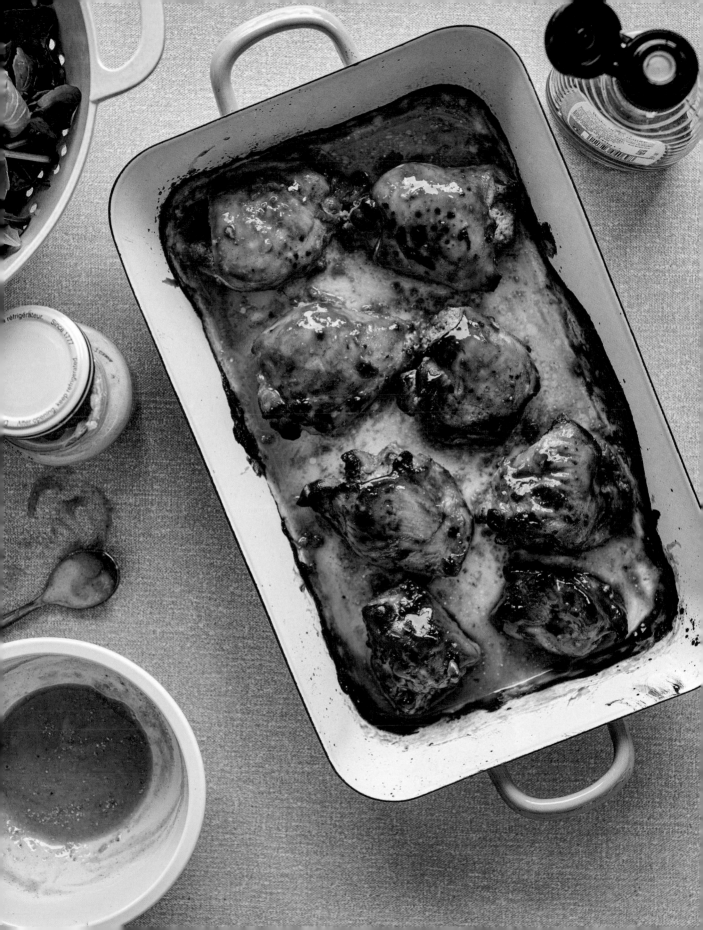

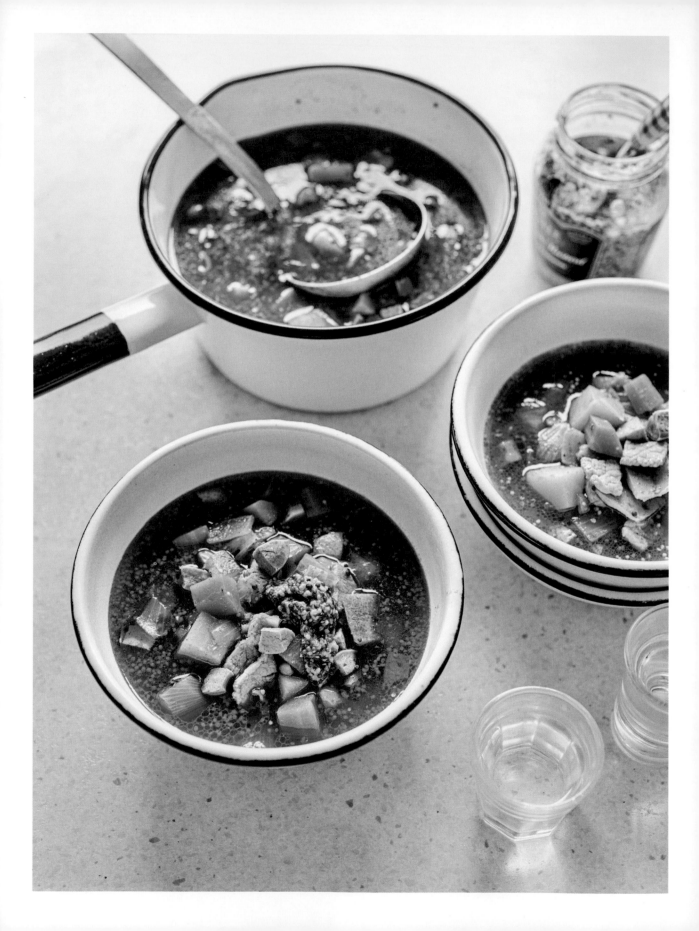

CHERNOBYL SOUP

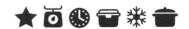

SERVES: 4
PREP: 5 minutes
COOK: 15 minutes
CALORIES: 338

This recipe is a modern classic from our blog, reported from one of our jollies – this time a glorious weekend in Ukraine, which included a full day exploring Chernobyl and the surrounding area. The soup is based on a simple broth that we were served inside the Chernobyl power plant, hence the name.

I can't recommend the Chernobyl tour enough: it's all very safe and well done but is a fascinating look into how close we all came to utter disaster. Mind, I've sat downwind of Paul after two bowlfuls of our chicken achari – I've stared into a poisonous abyss more than is decent.

Kiev did provide an exhilarating chance to defend Paul's honour, though: some rotter outside the main train station tried to pickpocket his wallet and so I got to puff out my shoulders and knock him over. The moment was made all the more delicious by the fact he had a trained monkey on his shoulder, which made for a surreal stare-down.

Paul commented afterwards that I had been terribly brave and honestly, he's not wrong – but when something you love dearly is in danger, instinct takes over. No way was I losing the wallet.

The soup, then: it's a matter of moments whether you have a pressure cooker or not. The key is to buy a pre-chopped vegetable mix – it'll save you all the time in the world.

8 bacon medallions, diced
100g (3½oz) smoked sausage,
   finely diced
1 tsp smoked paprika
600g (1lb 5oz) vegetable soup mix
   (pre-chopped swede, potato,
   onion, carrot)
1 litre (1¾ pints) vegetable stock
1 tbsp wholegrain mustard

Press the 'sauté' button on your pressure cooker and spray the pan with a little oil.

Add the bacon and sausage, stir, then add the paprika and the vegetable soup mix and cook for about 5 minutes, stirring occasionally.

Add the stock and mustard to the pan, and cook on high pressure for 10 minutes.

When finished, release the pressure and serve.

NOTE

You'll find the vegetable soup mix in nearly all the big supermarkets, but if you can't, you can easily make it yourself. Just finely chop swede, potato, carrot and onion in whatever proportions you prefer.

ONE PAN

BALSAMIC CHICKEN

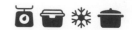

SERVES: 4
PREP: 10 minutes
COOK: 30 minutes
CALORIES: 235

Balsamic chicken is one of our go-to meals at Chubby Towers because it is ridiculously easy to prepare – and when we say prepare, really it amounts to nothing more than bumbling a few ingredients into the pan and stirring occasionally. All the best recipes are like this – there's certainly a time for me to be mincing around the kitchen with eight pans on the go and something fabulous in the oven, but I'm a lazy, lazy man, and this recipe speaks to me.

As an aside, can we talk vinegar for a moment? It'll certainly suit my acid tongue. When a recipe calls for vinegar, for the most part, you'll be absolutely fine with whatever is in the cupboard. However, when it's a key part of the dish, feel free to gussy it up with luxury brands. By way of example, we have a range of flavoured oils and vinegars that we use which we wouldn't be without, but they're saved for dishes like this or whacking a bit of extra flavour into salads.

This recipe, incidentally, works terribly well with noodles stirred through. But don't we all?

4 skinless, boneless chicken
   breasts
1 onion, finely diced
2 cloves of garlic, crushed
4 tbsp balsamic vinegar
600g (1lb 5oz) cherry tomatoes,
   halved
2 tsp dried rosemary
175ml (6fl oz) chicken stock
20g (¾oz) fresh basil leaves,
   chopped

Spray a large pan with a little oil and place it over a medium-high heat. Add the chicken and cook for 5–6 minutes each side, then remove from the pan and set aside.

Reduce the heat to medium, add the onion and garlic and cook for another 5 minutes. Add the balsamic vinegar to deglaze the pan, and cook until thickened.

Add the tomatoes, dried rosemary and stock and bring to the boil, then reduce the heat and simmer for 8–10 minutes.

Put the chicken back into the pan and gently stir into the sauce.

Serve, sprinkled with the chopped basil.

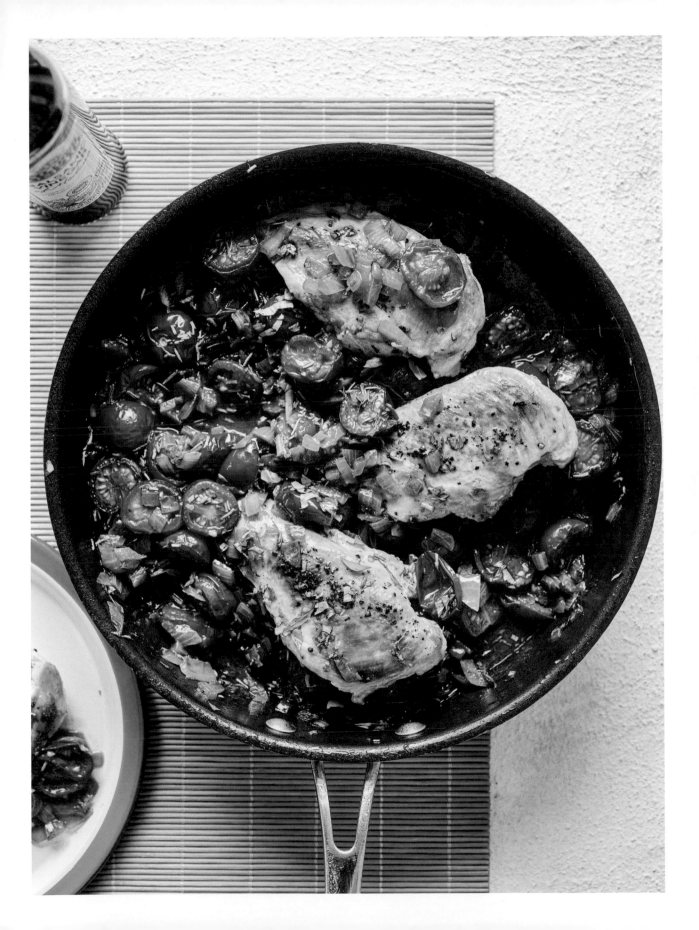

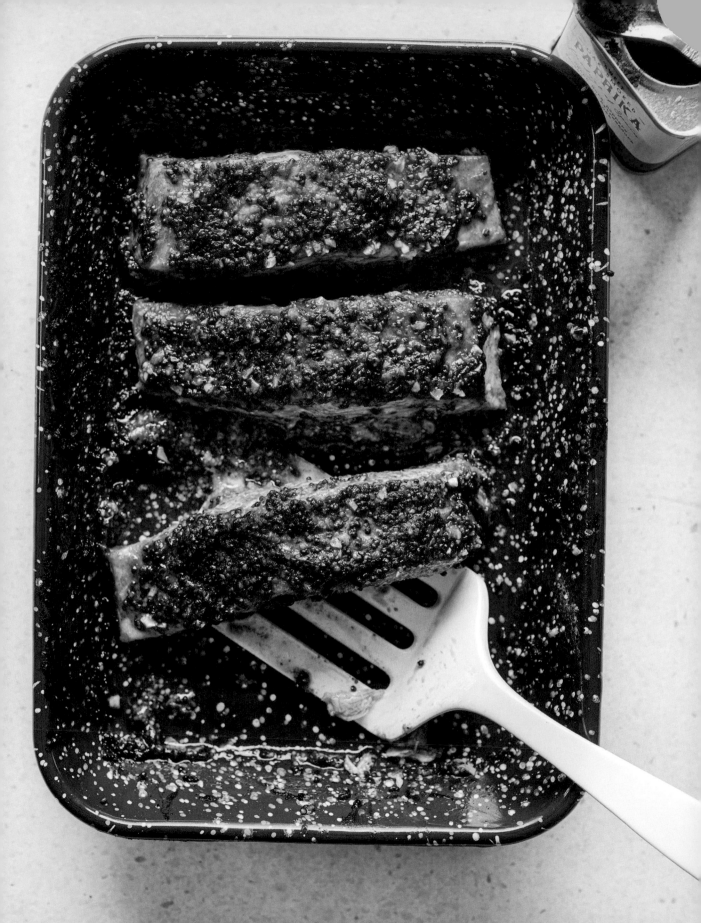

HONEY & MUSTARD SALMON

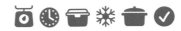

SERVES: 4
PREP: 5 minutes
COOK: 25 minutes
CALORIES: 386
DIET: GF/DF

Another doddle recipe, as we call them – make the sauce, marinate the fish and bang it in the oven. At the time of writing, we're holed up in a hotel and have been taking advantage of the room service menu – the star of which is this salmon. I asked for the recipe and we have changed it slightly to make it more friendly for your waistline. We care.

Living in a hotel does have its downsides, and not just as I slowly turn into Alan Partridge (though spare a thought for me, because that means Paul will turn into Lynne, his put-upon assistant – works though, doesn't it). I write during the day while Paul goes and picks up the bacon and well, sometimes you forget where you are.

Imagine me then, sitting writing at the desk with my earbuds in. Sitting in my most comfy, most tattered underwear, not a care in the world. 'Memory' from *Cats* came on and naturally that's my cue with the theatrical arm movements and imagined singing. I thought I was glorious – the housekeeper who had let herself in presuming the room was empty, less so.

Mind, we both hit the perfect high note with our screams. Rumour is that she has been signed off work, the sight of a pirouetting, hairy Bella Emberg etched forever in her mind.

3 tbsp wholegrain mustard
4 tsp honey
4 cloves of garlic, crushed
1 tsp smoked paprika
½ tsp cayenne pepper
½ tsp black pepper
4 salmon fillets

Preheat the oven to 180°C fan/400°F/gas mark 6.

Mix together the mustard, honey, garlic, paprika, cayenne and black pepper.

Spray an ovenproof dish with a little oil and place the salmon in it.

Using a spatula, spread the honey and mustard mixture over the salmon. Cover with foil and bake in the oven for 15–20 minutes.

Remove the foil and preheat the grill to medium-high.

Cook the salmon under the grill for 2–3 minutes.

Serve.

NOTE

We usually serve these with wedges, sautéed sugarsnap peas or grilled asparagus.

EGG FOO YUNG

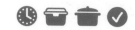

SERVES: 4
PREP: 5 minutes
COOK: 10 minutes
CALORIES: 100
DIET: VEG/DF

This eggy little treat is a staple in our Chinese takeaway orders, even though it requires zero skill to make and honestly can be made with ingredients you are bound to have in the cupboard. I've been eating this since I was a child, presumably because it was the cheapest item on the menu whenever Mother was too tired/drunk to make tea and had to order in.

My poor mother gets a bad reputation on the blog – anyone reading it may envision some harsh-faced shrew, with a fag permanently in the corner of her scowl and a bellicose, heartless attitude to life. That's unfair, because we've made no mention of the fact she's normally got a bottle of something in the other hand.

I jest: I've said it before, I couldn't wish for a better mother, and I know just the mere mention of her in here will raise a smile. What it will not raise is a few extra quid for me because she flatly refused to buy our first book, demanding a free copy instead. I promised her then that I would publicly shame her in the sequel, and so here we are.

Paul's mother exists.

Speaking of eggy beasts, the egg foo yung – it can handle all sorts of extras. Chopped ham and peppers are particular favourites of ours.

4 large eggs, beaten
60g (2¼oz) beansprouts
2 spring onions, finely sliced
½ tsp sesame oil
1 tsp oyster sauce
2 tsp light or dark soy sauce
1 tsp rice wine vinegar

Mix everything together in a bowl and stir.

Spray a small frying pan with a little oil and place over a high heat.

Pour the mix into the pan and use a spoon or spatula to drag the beansprouts to the middle as best you can, ensuring that they cook fully.

Leave to cook for about 3–4 minutes, then flip over.

Cook for another 3 minutes, then serve.

NOTE

This is champion with some rice, or as a side to other Chinese dishes.

ONE PAN

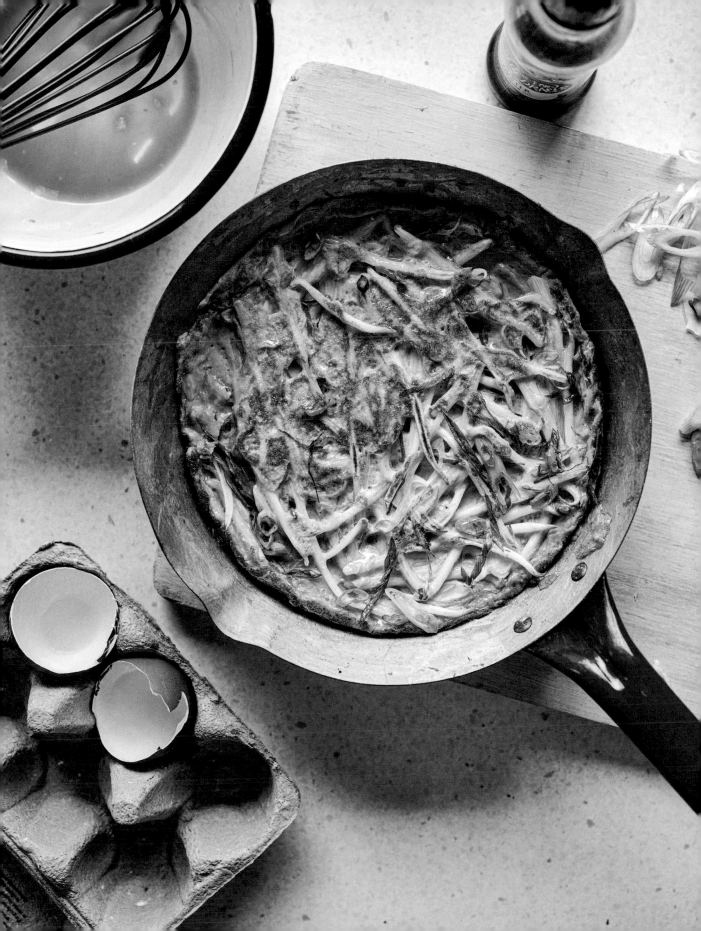

LIL' ONION CURRY

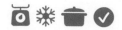

SERVES: 4
PREP: 10 minutes
COOK: 35 minutes
CALORIES: 355
DIET: GF/DF

Paul is insisting on the 'lil' in the title and between this and the 'fam' earlier in the book, I truly don't know what has come over him. Certainly won't be me if he carries on like this, I assure you.

However, we can forgive him his foray into speaking like he's a member of Grazin' Squad because this curry is a joyous occasion. According to him, he only added the chopped-up pickled onions because he had grown tired of the 800 or so half-empty jars that were rattling around in the fridge. We'll let him have that one, and I'll let him know what I'm tired of later when you go to bed.

As an aside, naan breads are a doddle to make if you have self-raising flour and yoghurt in the house. We don't measure, but generally go for a ratio of three-quarters flour to yoghurt. Knead until it's come together, shape into balls, smash down and fry in a hot pan.

1 tsp ground turmeric
4 skinless, boneless chicken breasts, diced
2 tsp fennel seeds
1 × 440g (16oz) jar of baby silverskin onions, drained and roughly chopped
4 green chillies, deseeded and chopped
2 bay leaves
4 cloves of garlic, crushed
8cm (3 inches) ginger, grated
1½ tbsp ground coriander
1 tbsp light brown sugar
160ml (5½fl oz) coconut cream
2 tsp hot chilli powder
a pinch of salt
4 tbsp chopped fresh coriander

Sprinkle the turmeric over the chicken and toss.

Spray a large pan with a little oil and place it over a medium-high heat. Add the fennel seeds and stir round the pan for about 30 seconds.

Add the pickled onions, green chillies and bay leaves and stir well for 2 minutes, then add the garlic and ginger and stir again.

Add the chicken and the ground coriander to the pan along with 120ml (4fl oz) of water and the sugar, and stir well. Reduce the heat to medium-low, cover the pan with a lid, and cook for 15 minutes.

Add the coconut cream, chilli powder and a pinch of salt and cook for another 10 minutes with the lid on.

Remove the bay leaves and serve topped with the chopped coriander.

NOTES

This will give a good tang! If that's not for you, simply rinse the onions in a sieve before chopping them.

Serve with rice.

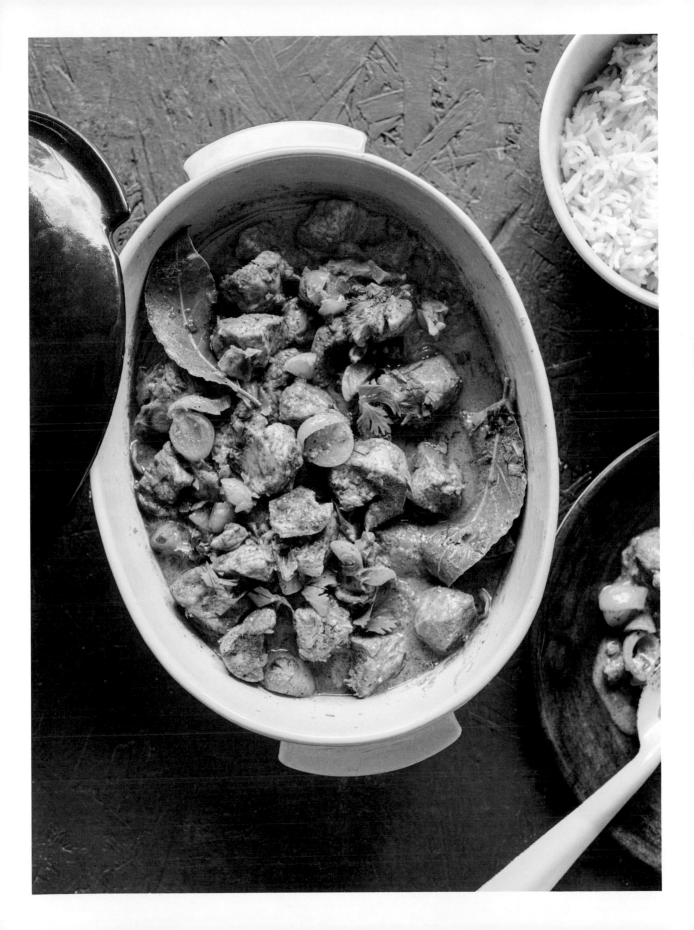

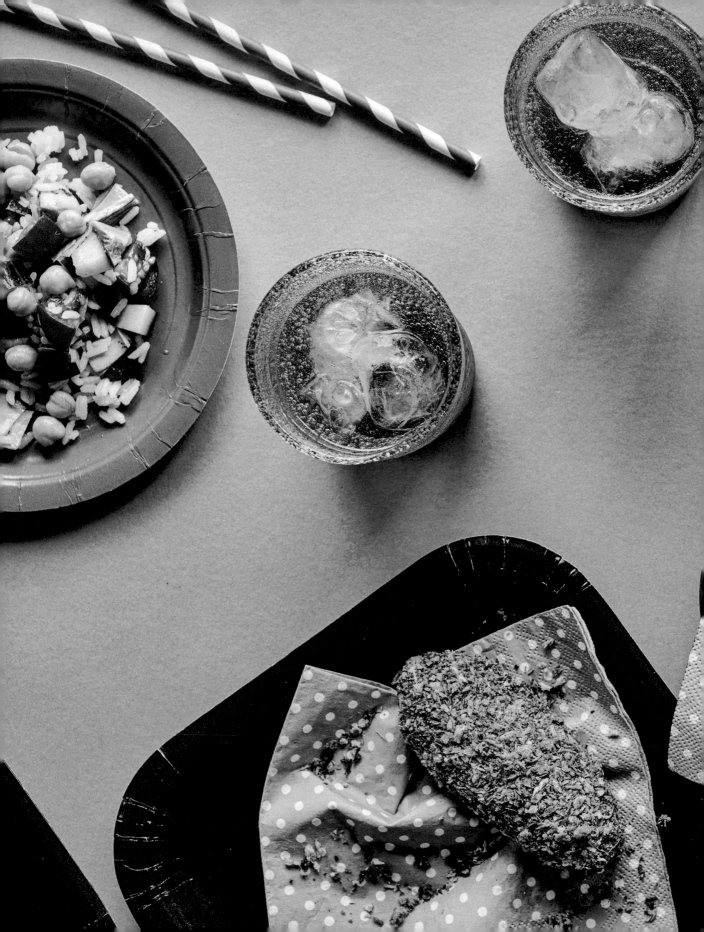

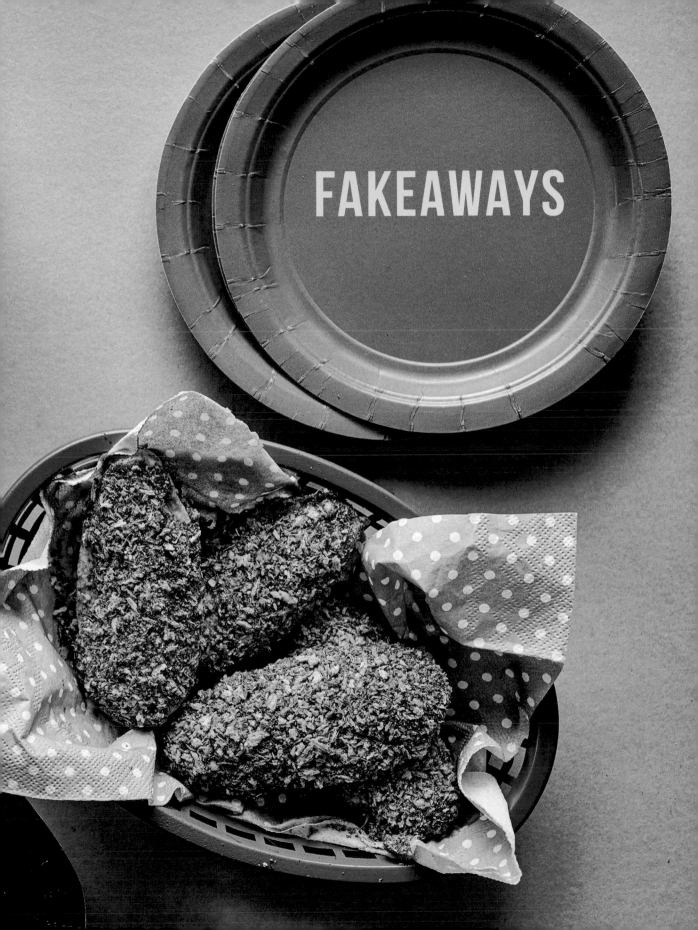

FAKEAWAYS

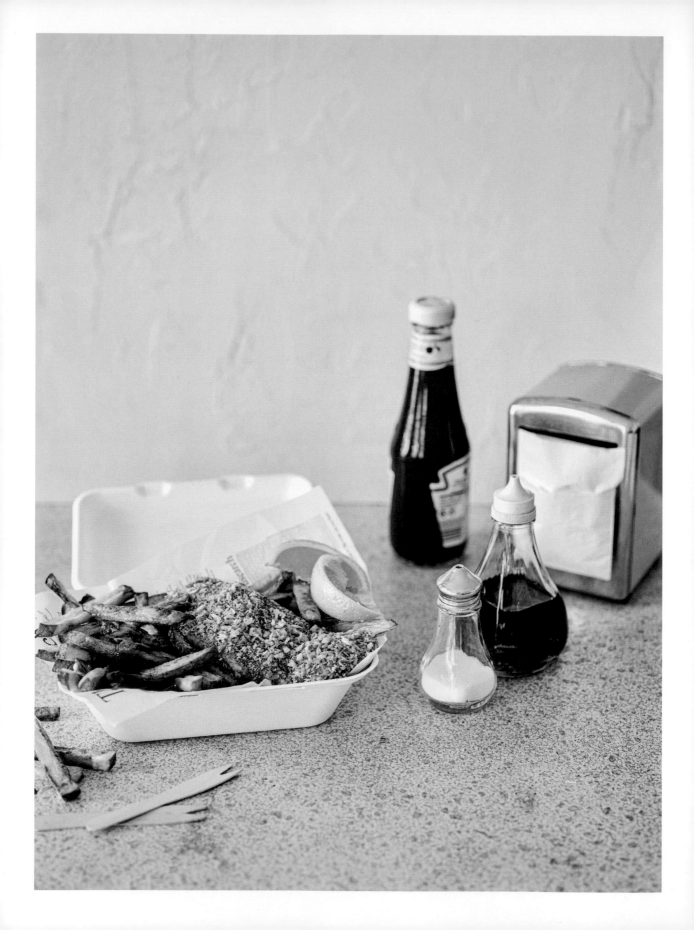

EASY FISH 'N' CHIPS

SERVES: 4
PREP: 10 minutes
COOK: 40 minutes
CALORIES: 431
DIET: DF

As this is a wonderfully simple recipe, we are going to include a couple of extra 'side' ideas in the notes, so do make sure you take a look. This is a slimming take on fish and chips which (although it eschews the delicious batter that we all know, love and would put someone through a plate glass window for) hits the spot.

Settle an argument for us, though. Paul insists on this weird gloop on the side called 'pink sauce'. To me, it's ketchup and mayonnaise combined in one frightfully manky sauce. He reckons it's a culinary masterpiece. Clearly he's wrong, but please do feel free to get in touch via social media to tell him that.

Mind, if you're someone who thinks a pea wet is delicious, we don't want to hear from you at all. Because you're clearly a pervert.

900g (2lb) potatoes
4 cod fillets
2 eggs, beaten
60g (2¼oz) panko breadcrumbs
1 lemon, quartered

Preheat the oven to 220°C fan/475°F/gas mark 9.

Wash the potatoes and slice into chips.

Spray them with oil and spread them on a baking tray, then bake in the oven for 40 minutes, turning halfway (or even better, cook in an air fryer).

Meanwhile, gently dip the fish into the beaten eggs and then into the breadcrumbs until well coated.

Bake in the oven for 8–10 minutes, then finish under the grill on a medium-high heat for 2–3 minutes to get them golden.

Divide the fish and chips between four plates, squeeze over the lemon wedges and serve.

NOTES

Making your own mushy peas is a matter of moments and well worth the time if you're a fan, but if you're making a quick dinner, take a normal can of mushy peas, add a sliver of butter (trust us) and a teaspoon of mint sauce.

Paul likes to make pink sauce to go with his dinner. Mix half tomato ketchup with light mayonnaise. Add a touch of smoked paprika and a pinch of sea salt.

I'm a curry sauce man but recommend the Mayflower curry sauce you can buy from most discount food shops. It tastes exactly like a chippy sauce.

Chippy dinners aren't the same without a pickled egg. If you have a look on our blog, we have a fabulous recipe for eggs pickled in beetroot vinegar. Absolutely worth a look!

SMART SWAP

Any white fish will do for this – haddock and pollock are great alternatives.

QUICK KATSU

SERVES: 4
PREP: 15 minutes
COOK: 35 minutes
CALORIES: 438

We have been meaning to create a quick 'katsu' recipe for an age, but I shan't lie: it's been an absolute ball-ache. Me and my delicate phrasing, I know. We have gone through about ten different iterations before getting something we're happy with, and we present it below.

Chicken katsu is my go-to dish in the more popular chains – you know, those places where the dishes come round on individually coloured plates? Terrific idea until you turn up with someone with an entirely missing sense of self-restraint and a lax attitude to spending other people's money. We motored our way through plate after plate until I could barely see my friend behind what looked like a Pride plate tribute to the Leaning Tower of Pisa and had to call it a day. Luckily our gorging had managed to fall on the one day of the year they remembered their wallet, otherwise I'd still be doing shifts in the kitchen to make up the bill.

A quick note on the sauce: it does look a little bit like a slick of meconium, but I beg of you to look past that. It is delicious.

4 skinless, boneless chicken breasts
3 eggs, beaten
70g (2½oz) panko breadcrumbs
2 onions, finely diced
4 cloves of garlic, crushed
4cm (1½ inches) ginger, finely grated
2 tsp ground turmeric
4 tbsp mild curry powder
1 tsp chilli flakes
2 tbsp plain flour
600ml (20fl oz) chicken stock
2 tsp light soy sauce
150ml (5fl oz) coconut milk
½ tsp honey

Preheat the oven to 200°C fan/425°F/gas mark 7.

Dip each chicken breast in the beaten egg and toss in the breadcrumbs to coat, patting on some extra breadcrumbs to any bits where they didn't stick.

Lay the chicken on a baking sheet and cook in the oven for 20 minutes.

Meanwhile, spray a saucepan with a little oil and place it over a medium heat.

Add the onions, garlic and ginger to the pan and fry until softened, then add all the spices and cook for another 2 minutes, stirring frequently.

Add the flour and give it a good stir, then slowly add the chicken stock to the pan, stirring continuously until well mixed.

Add the soy sauce and coconut milk and stir, and finally add the honey.

Remove from the heat and leave to cool a bit, then blend with a stick blender (or use a food processor).

Serve the chicken with the sauce poured over.

NOTE

Serve with rice.

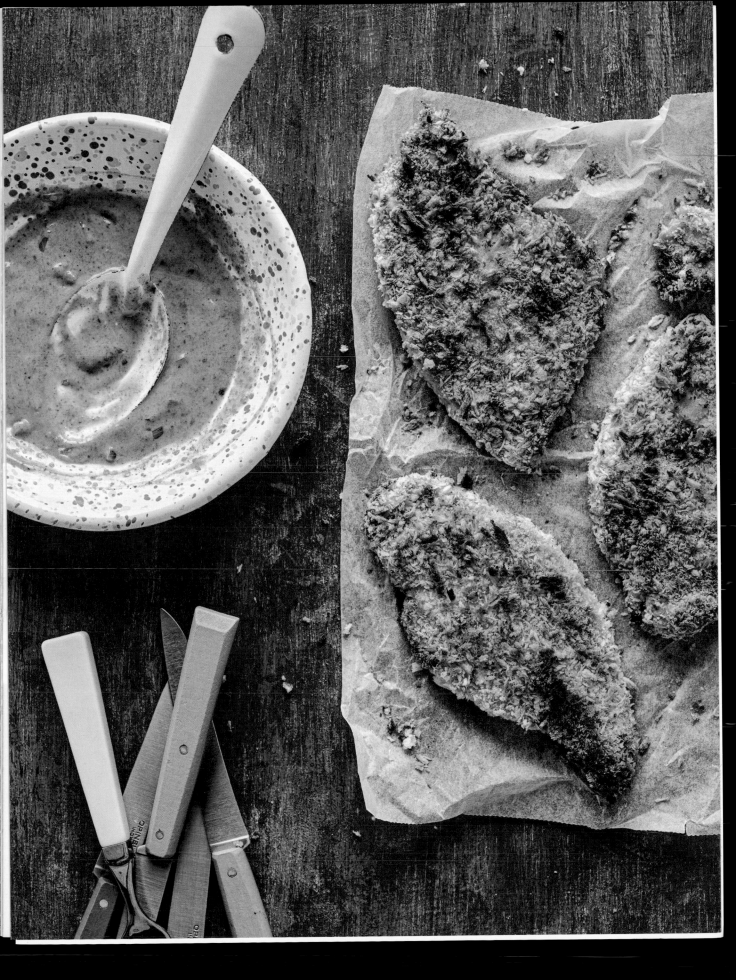

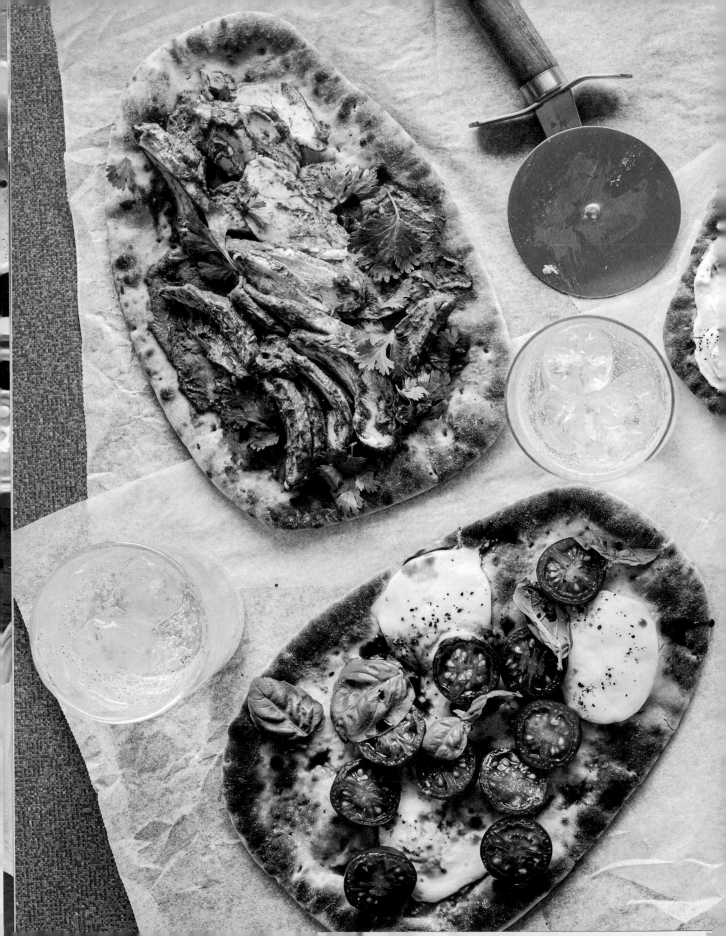

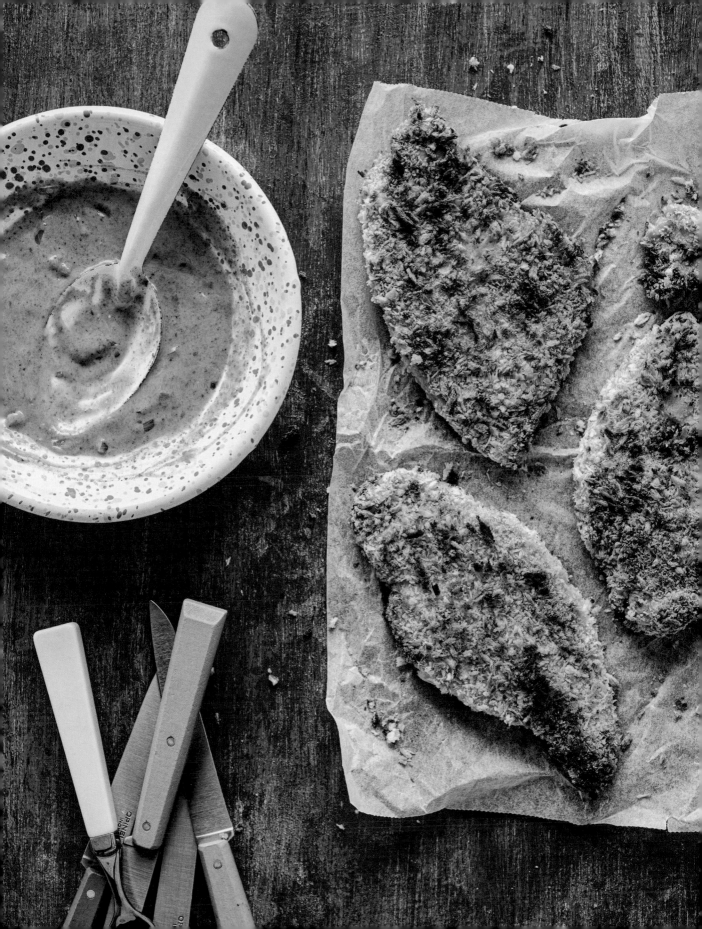

GREEK BURGERS

SERVES: 4
PREP: 10 minutes
COOK: 15 minutes
CALORIES: 446

You've noticed, surely, that we're huge fans of burgers and have done almost every conceivable variation of the buggers since we started writing. As a friend, who will remain nameless (Gary J. Main, Hebburn, early forties), once said, 'There's something reassuring and wholesome about juicy meat slipped between your buns'. You know I'm right, of course. And no – we're absolutely not above slipping a friend's name into our cookbook purely to have a shot at getting in his knickers. Mind, 20 Benson & Hedges and a Wham bar has the same unlocking effect.

Anyway, we digress, as ever. The tzatziki suggested really makes the dish, but if you can't be fussed shop-bought will be tickety-boo, though understandably higher in calories. Why does everything that tastes so good betray us so?

For the burgers
500g (1lb 2oz) lean lamb mince
4 wholemeal buns, sliced
4 handfuls of lettuce leaves
½ red onion, sliced
2 large tomatoes, sliced
¼ cucumber, sliced

For the tzatziki
6 tbsp fat-free Greek yoghurt
¼ cucumber, deseeded and
　the flesh and skin grated
juice of ½ lemon
¼ tsp dried dill
1 clove garlic, crushed
20g (¾oz) reduced-fat feta
　cheese, crumbled
1 tsp mint sauce
a pinch of salt

Preheat the grill to medium-high.

Mix the tzatziki ingredients together in a bowl, then cover with clingfilm and pop into the fridge.

Gently work the lamb mince together in a bowl with your hands, then divide into four.

Take each lump of mince and roll it into a ball, then flatten into a burger shape.

Put the burgers under the grill and cook on each side for about 6–8 minutes until cooked through.

Place the burgers in the buns and top with a dollop of tzatziki, the lettuce, onion, tomatoes and sliced cucumber.

NOTE
To deseed a cucumber, simply cut it in half lengthways and scoop out the soft centre with a teaspoon.

SMART SWAP
You can also use lean beef mince for this – if you do, it's best to divide the mixture into eight (so there's two in each bun), just to prevent them being too dry.

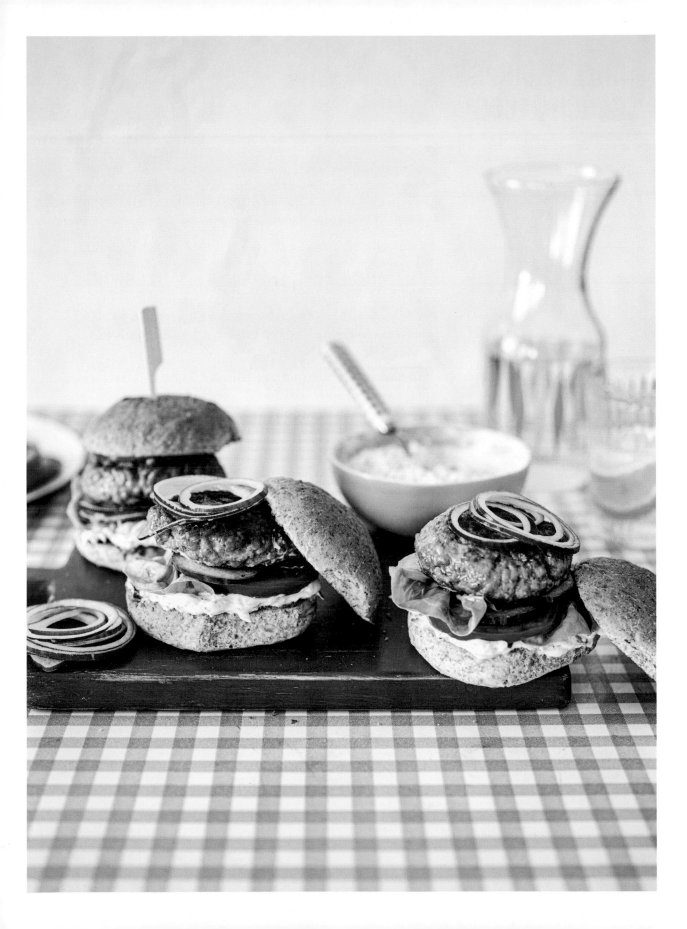

CHEESY CHIPS WITH HOMEMADE RANCH SAUCE

SERVES: 4
PREP: 10 minutes
COOK: 45 minutes
CALORIES: 320
DIET: VEG/GF
(check cheese is vegetarian friendly)

I don't know about you, but someone could hook me up to some dodgy medical equipment, transfuse my rubbish glittery blood with neat ranch dressing, and I'd sit up and thank them afterwards before collapsing into a happy, garlicky mess.

The first time Paul and I went to Florida for a fortnight at Disney, we were wandering around a mall and stopped at what we thought was a fancy restaurant in a desperate need of salad and vitamins. I spooned ranch dressing on without knowing what it was (I didn't have my glasses on so probably presumed it was raunch dressing, and I am all for that).

Well: I don't know if it was delirium from the heat or having my head knocked silly on the Incredible Hulk rollercoaster, but that was very much a turning point in my life. Some folks think of keystone dates as when they got married or had children. My epiphany was garlic mayo in what was the equivalent of a Harvester restaurant.

Still, we're all our own people. If you had the time, inclination and the courage/foolhardiness to risk the wrath/mooing of the author of the emotional support potatoes from the previous book, the ranch dressing pairs up very nicely with those too.

4 large potatoes
½ tsp paprika
1 tsp garlic granules
125g (4½oz) fat-free Greek yoghurt
2 cloves of garlic, crushed
½ tsp dried dill
½ tsp lemon juice
a pinch of salt and black pepper
160g (5¾oz) reduced-fat cheese, grated
a handful of fresh chives, chopped

Preheat the oven to 220°C fan/475°F/gas mark 9.

Cut the potatoes into chips and coat them with the paprika and garlic granules. Spray them with oil and spread them on a baking tray, then bake in the oven for 40 minutes, turning halfway (or even better, cook in an air fryer).

Meanwhile, mix together the yoghurt, garlic, dill, lemon juice, salt and pepper to make the ranch sauce, and set aside.

When the chips are cooked, top them with the cheese and put them back into the oven for another 4–5 minutes.

Remove from the oven, drizzle with the ranch sauce and top with the chives.

> **NOTE**
> The best cheeses to use for this are mozzarella, Cheddar or Red Leicester.

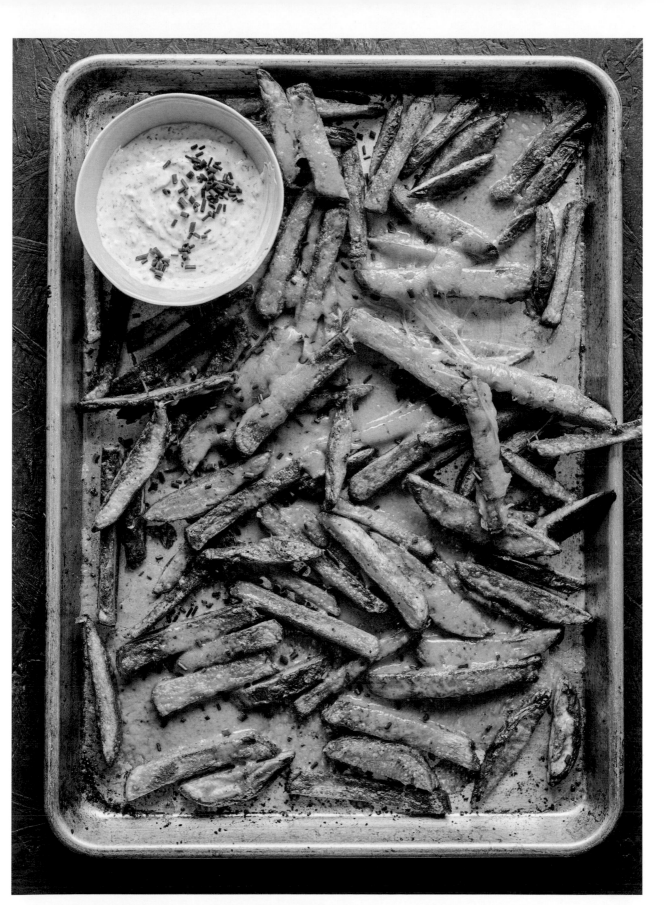

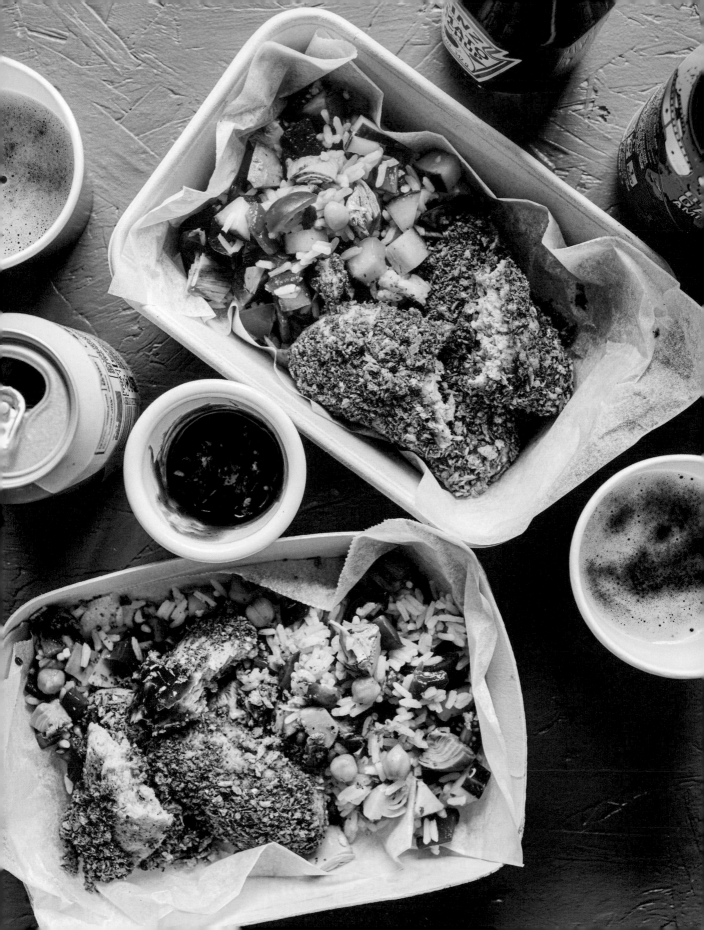

SOUTHERN-FRIED(ESQUE) FAUX CHICKEN RICE BOX

SERVES: 4
PREP: 15 minutes
COOK: 40 minutes
CALORIES: 496
DIET: VEG/DF

2 eggs, beaten
4 Quorn fillets, defrosted

For the flavoured breadcrumbs
75g (3oz) panko breadcrumbs
2 tbsp onion granules
1 tbsp salt
1 tbsp black pepper
1 tbsp garlic granules
1 tbsp dried thyme
1 tbsp dried sage
1 tbsp dried marjoram
1 tbsp dried mixed herbs
1 tbsp ground ginger
1 tbsp paprika
1 tbsp mustard powder
1 tbsp cayenne pepper

For the rice
175g (6oz) long-grain rice
½ cucumber, deseeded and
    chopped
50g (2oz) marinated artichokes,
    chopped
300g (10½oz) cherry tomatoes,
    diced
75g (3oz) roasted red peppers,
    chopped
1 × 400g (14oz) tin of chickpeas,
    drained and rinsed

There's no time for a flashy intro here: let me just tell you the facts. This recipe uses our chubby bakes chicken but in a flash of genius turns it into a more substantial dinner by 'paying homage' to the popular rice-box from a well-known chain. Quorn fillets work wonderfully here, but feel free to stick with chicken.

Preheat the oven to 200°C fan/425°F/gas mark 7.

Mix together all the ingredients for the flavoured breadcrumbs in a shallow dish. Put the beaten eggs into another dish.

Dip the fillets in the beaten egg, allow any excess to drip off, then gently roll in the flavoured breadcrumbs.

Lay the chicken on a baking sheet and bake for 35–40 minutes.

Meanwhile, cook the rice according to the packet instructions, then drain.

Put the rest of the rice ingredients into a bowl, mix with the rice, and serve, topped with the chicken.

NOTES

To make this even speedier, you could use microwave pouches of rice. You'll need half a pouch per person.

We quite like having BBQ sauce on the side with this one.

SMART SWAPS

Can't be chewed on with all those herbs and spices? Don't worry – just use whatever seasoning you have!

The roasted red peppers are the ones in the jar. If you can't find them, a standard red pepper will do.

There's a cracking recipe for 'takeaway' baked beans on our blog!

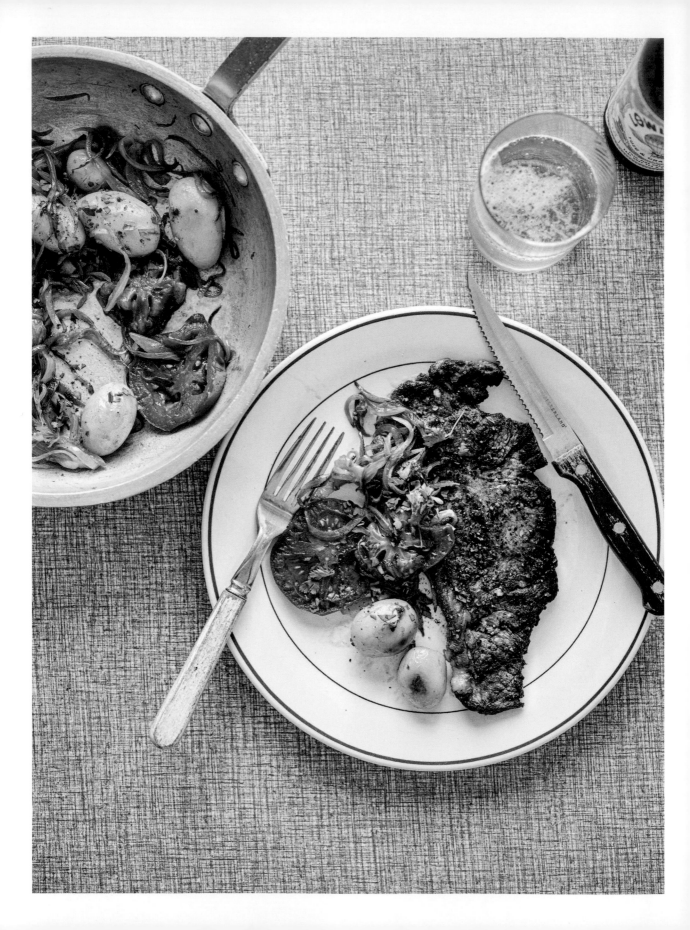

SPECIAL STEAK DINNER

SERVES: 1
PREP: 5 minutes
COOK: 20 minutes
CALORIES: 476
DIET: GF

We got the idea to include this recipe in response to – steak and BJ day, which is celebrated a month after Valentine's Day and is well, exactly as you ought to imagine. We're big fans of both, though at my age I'd rather just have two steaks if I'm honest. In the spirit of being inclusive to all our readers, we've made this a lovely dish for one, but of course it can be scaled up as appropriate.

Paul suggests serving this meal wrapped up in a hedge-fresh copy of *Salsa* magazine, which he assures me was his reading material of choice way back when. No such luxury for me – I had to make do with a 28.8k dial-up connection and a whole lot of patience: nothing worse than being at Billy Mill roundabout (google it) only to lose your connection because your mum is feverishly trying to get on Richard & Judy's *You Say We Pay*. Sigh.

1 × 300g (10½oz) tin of new
    potatoes, drained
¼ tsp paprika
1 steak of your choice
1 onion, sliced
1 tomato, sliced
2 tsp butter
1 tbsp chopped fresh coriander

Preheat the oven to 200°C fan/425°F/gas mark 7.

Halve the potatoes, sprinkle with the paprika and set aside.

Heat a large ovenproof frying pan over a high heat and spray it with a little oil. Add the steak, onion, tomato and potatoes, each in its own quarter of the pan, and cook for 1–2 minutes.

Flip the steak and place the butter on top, then cook for another minute, spooning some of the juice from the pan over the veg.

Place the pan in the oven for 4–6 minutes, then remove and leave to rest for 10 minutes.

Sprinkle with the coriander and serve.

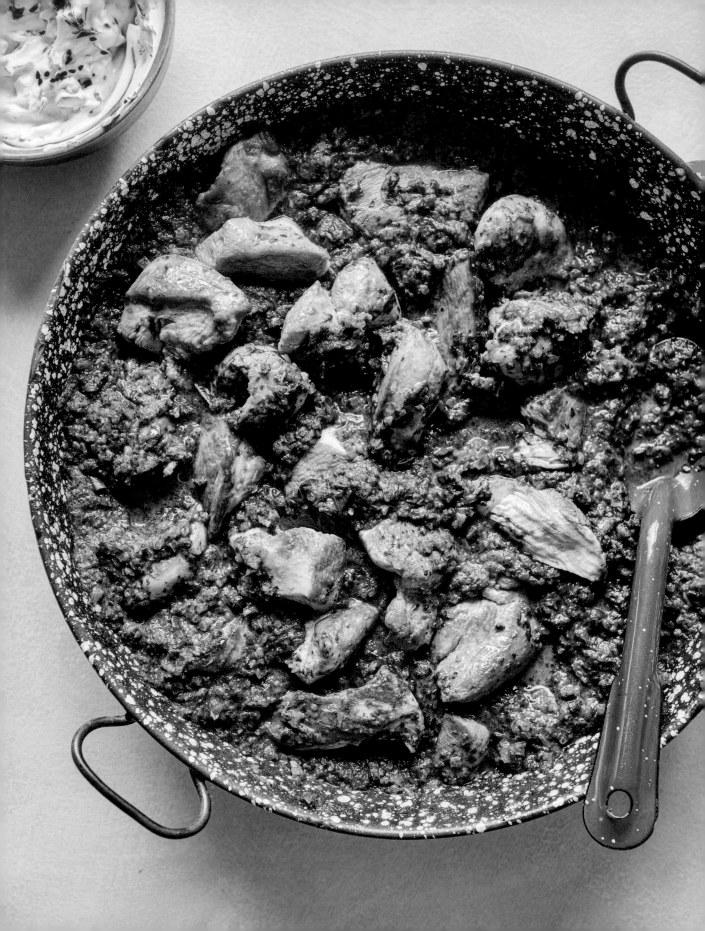

CHICKEN TIKKA SAAG

SERVES: 4
PREP: 10 minutes
COOK: 25 minutes
CALORIES: 253

Just look at this, will you? It's absolutely and utterly delicious. If you're not a fan of spinach then yes, you may be on a sticky wicket with this one, but the combination of spices and flavourings really makes this dish come alive. You could bulk it out by adding some softly boiled potato if you wanted a more substantial dish, but this – mixed with rice and slathered on a naan – will never let you down.

I should say – do remember that you've had this dish when it comes to the day after. Without wanting to be gross, it does have the effect of turning your excretions a startling green colour. I'm sorry to mention it, but being a hypochondriac, I do notice these things. You should have seen my panic after I overdid the beetroot salad from page 205 – I was on the phone to 111 for a good twenty minutes before I realized my error.

2 tsp ground cumin
2 tsp ground coriander
2 tsp garam masala
1 tsp ground turmeric
½ tsp mild chilli powder
2 onions, finely diced
3 cloves of garlic, crushed
6cm (2½ inches) ginger, grated
260g (9oz) frozen spinach
250ml (9fl oz) chicken stock
200g (7fl oz) passata
4 skinless, boneless chicken
    breasts, diced

Mix together the cumin, coriander, garam masala, turmeric and chilli powder and set aside.

Spray a large frying pan with a little oil and place it over a medium heat. Add the onions and cook for 3 minutes, stirring frequently.

Add the garlic and ginger to the pan along with the spice mix and cook for 1 minute, stirring constantly.

Add the spinach, stock and passata and cook for another 5 minutes. Remove from the heat and leave to cool for a few minutes, then blend with a stick blender.

Spray another pan with a little oil and place it over a medium-high heat. Add the chicken and cook for 5–6 minutes, making sure no pink remains.

Reduce the heat to medium, add the sauce to the pan and bring to a simmer for 5 minutes.

Serve.

NOTE

Serve with rice.

5 TOPPED NAAN BREADS

The idea for topped naan breads came to me in a flash of bewilderingly loud inspiration, in the form of having them thrust in front of my face at the end of a long, long day by an overly animated friend. Stroking his ego is always a dangerous business, but they were delicious.

The naan bread might seem like a doughy slice of no when you're on a diet, but give them a go as a base – they're really not terrible in terms of calories.

That said, if you do fancy switching things up, all the suggestions below will happily top a potato.

SERVES: 2
PREP: 5 minutes
COOK: 0 minutes
CALORIES: 443

CHICKEN TIKKA

100g (3½oz) cooked chicken, chopped
½ tsp garam masala
½ tsp chilli powder
¼ tsp ground cumin
¼ tsp paprika
¼ tsp ground turmeric
⅛ tsp ground coriander
1 tbsp fat-free natural yoghurt
1 tbsp mayonnaise
1 tsp tomato purée
1 warm naan bread
fresh coriander leaves (optional)

Mix everything except the coriander leaves together in a bowl and spread out over a naan bread.

Garnish with coriander leaves, if you like.

SERVES: 2
PREP: 5 minutes
COOK: 0 minutes
CALORIES: 324

HAWAIIAN

2 tbsp extra-light soft cheese
1 warm naan bread
2 slices of prosciutto, torn up
1 pineapple ring, cut into wedges

Spread the soft cheese over a naan bread and top with the prosciutto and pineapple.

SERVES: 2
PREP: 5 minutes
COOK: 0 minutes
CALORIES: 317

MEDITERRANEAN SALAD

1 warm naan bread
80g (3oz) tin of tuna chunks, drained
3 cherry tomatoes, halved
1 tsp capers
1 tbsp feta, crumbled feta cheese
¼ red onion, sliced
1 tsp balsamic vinegar

Top a naan bread with all the ingredients and drizzle over the balsamic vinegar.

SERVES: 2
PREP: 5 minutes
COOK: 5 minutes
CALORIES: 321
DIET: VEG (check mozzarella is vegetarian friendly)

JUICY TOMATO CAPRESE

1 naan bread
50g (1¾oz) mozzarella cheese, cut into
    chunks
3 cherry tomatoes, halved
2 tbsp balsamic vinegar
4 fresh basil leaves

Top a naan bread with the mozzarella and cherry tomatoes and pop under a hot grill for a few minutes.

Remove from the grill, drizzle with the balsamic vinegar, and top with the basil leaves.

SERVES: 2
PREP: 5 minutes
COOK: 5 minutes
CALORIES: 318
DIET: VEG (check mozzarella is vegetarian friendly)

CHEESY PIZZA

1 tbsp tomato purée
1 clove of garlic, crushed
1 naan bread
50g (1¾oz) mozzarella cheese, grated
1 tomato, sliced
4 fresh basil leaves, sliced

Mix together the tomato purée and garlic, and spread over a naan bread.

Top with the mozzarella and tomato and place under a hot grill for a few minutes.

Remove from the heat and sprinkle over the sliced basil.

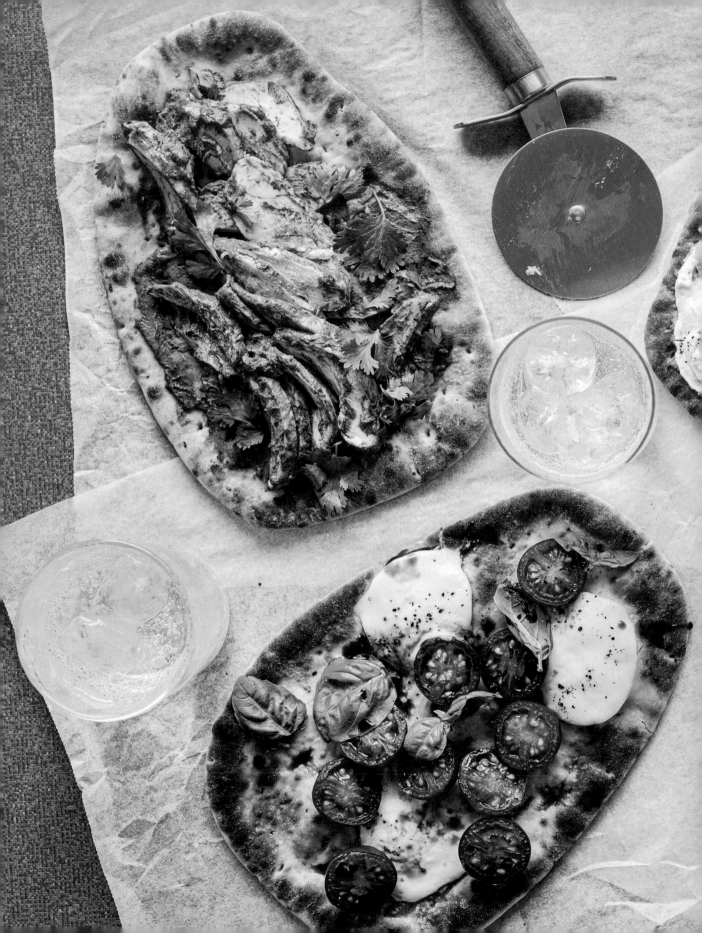

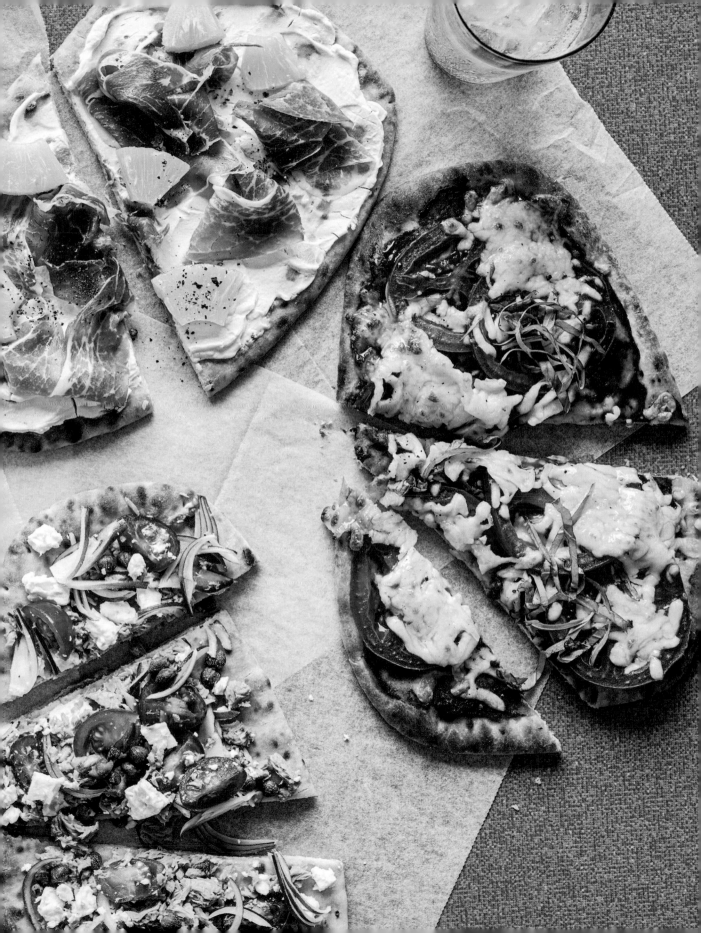

CHICKEN YAKITORI

SERVES: 4
PREP: 20 minutes
COOK: 35 minutes
CALORIES: 346
DIET: DF

I shall start this intro with a gentle recommendation and a bit of health and safety: when you're using skewers, you must always assume they're trying to kill you.

Metal skewers are designed for two purposes: to stab your fingers while you root around in the cutlery drawer trying to find them, or to sink through your flesh like a hot knife through butter when you forget the oven-mitts and try to turn them with your hand.

Wooden skewers are slightly less injurious, as long as you remember they're itching to burst into flame at a moment's notice. As someone who treats fire as an unexpected consequence to most things, I'm always surprised when I open the grill to find the skewers blazing away in an oven full of smoke. Heed Paul's tip in the notes. I suggest water rather than paraffin, but you do you.

400g (14oz) skinless, boneless chicken thighs
400g (14oz) skinless, boneless chicken breasts
80ml (2½fl oz) dark soy sauce
3 tbsp mirin
2 tbsp brown sugar
1 tbsp cider vinegar
1 tsp black pepper
4 cloves of garlic, crushed
5cm (2 inches) ginger, finely grated
1 tsp oil
2 spring onions, sliced

Dice the chicken into thin 3cm (1¼ inch) pieces and pop them into a bowl.

In another bowl, mix together the soy sauce, mirin, sugar and cider vinegar, along with 6 tablespoons of water.

Add the black pepper, garlic, ginger and oil to the chicken and mix well.

Spoon 4 tablespoons of the sauce on to the chicken, then toss well to mix.

Pour the rest of the sauce into a small pan and bring to the boil over a medium heat, then reduce to a simmer. Keep stirring for 10–15 minutes, until it has thickened.

Preheat the grill to medium-high.

Thread the chicken onto the skewers. Brush it with more sauce (don't be shy, really slather it on) and grill for 3–4 minutes.

Brush with yet more sauce, then turn and grill for another 3–4 minutes.

Serve with the spring onions sprinkled over the top.

NOTES

If using wooden skewers, make sure to soak them for 20 minutes first to prevent them from burning.

These work brilliantly on the barbecue too!

Serve with rice or noodles.

SMART SWAP

If you haven't got mirin, rice wine vinegar will do.

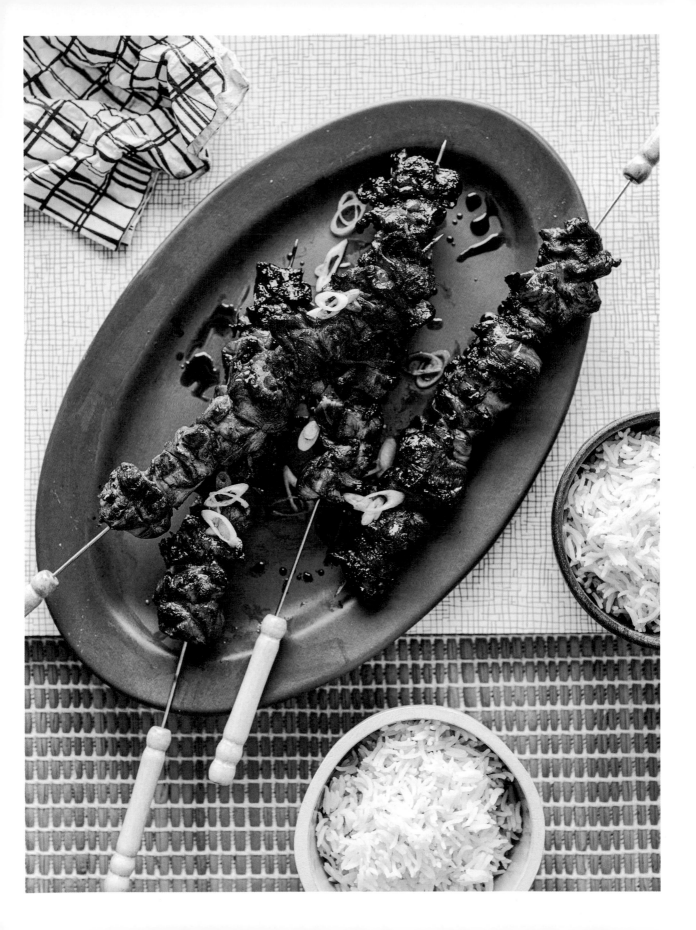

POUTINE (SORT OF)

SERVES: 4
PREP: 10 minutes
COOK: 40 minutes
CALORIES: 333

This is cheesy chips and gravy. We shan't gussy it up: it's a quick take on poutine, one of Canada's greatest dishes. You can top it with all sorts of excitement, but sometimes it is the purest form that works best of all.

I've already waxed lyrical about Canada, so instead, unbeknownst to Paul who thinks this is an introduction about chips, I'm going to tell you what he means to me. Paul gets so much schtick in my writing that you would be forgiven for thinking we existed in a marriage of convenience, spending our days throwing barbs at one another.

The truth is I catch myself looking at Paul, or thinking of the things we have done together, and falling in love anew. At the time of writing we have fallen asleep together over 5,000 times, and every morning I find myself appreciating the fact he's right there beside me, dribbling on the pillow like a tranquillized walrus and polluting the fresh morning air.

I am, forgive the schmaltz, an incredibly lucky man. To have a perfect other who can always make me laugh, who thinks nothing of himself and everything of me. I could wish for no better.

So, here's to Paul. The unsung hero. The quiet cub. The keystone upon which every part of my life is built and the support which keeps it all from falling quietly apart.

1kg (2lb 4oz) potatoes
125g (4½oz) mozzarella cheese, cut into small chunks
300ml (10fl oz) chicken gravy, heated up

Preheat the oven to 200°C fan/425°F/gas mark 7.

You know the drill for chips – cut the potatoes into chips, spray with oil and cook in the oven for 40 minutes, turning halfway – or even better, skip preheating the oven and cook them in an air fryer.

Serve the chips on plates and top with the diced mozzarella and a good drizzling of gravy.

NOTES

With sincere apologies to Canada. They usually use cheese curds in this but they're a bugger to get hold of in the UK – mozzarella is pretty close, which is what makes this 'sort of'.

Any standard white potato will do, but the best results will be with Maris Piper, King Edward or Marabel.

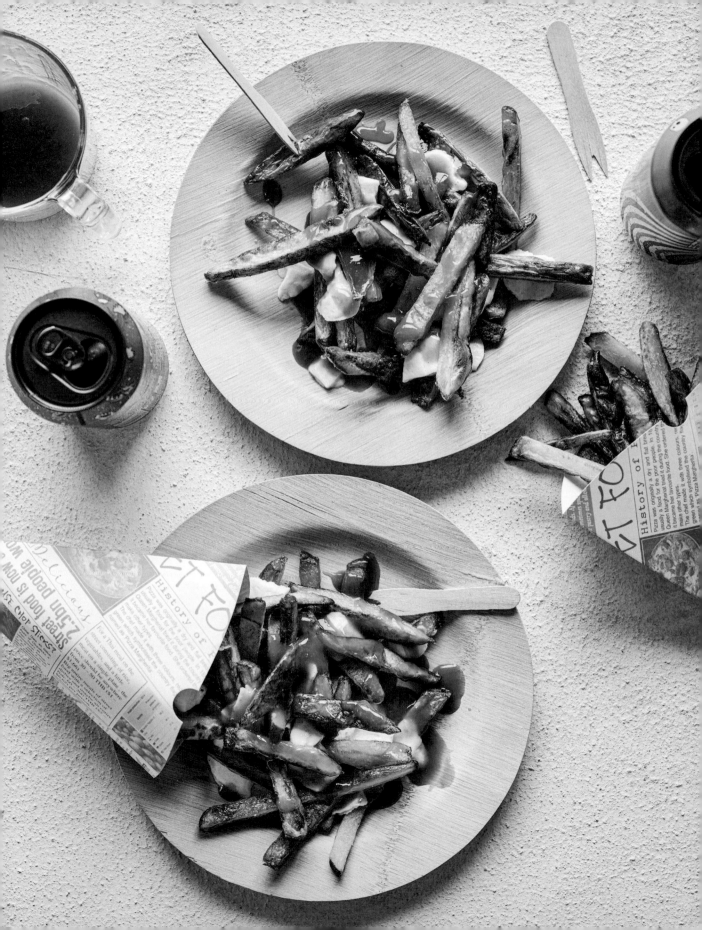

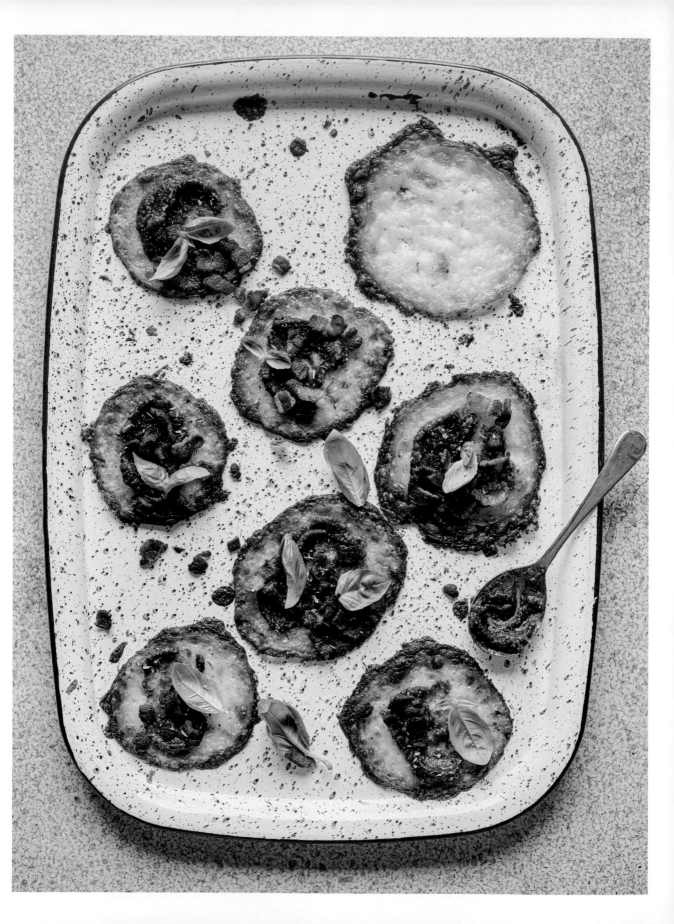

PIZZA DISCS

MAKES: 12
PREP: 5 minutes
COOK: 10 minutes
CALORIES: 57 calories per disc
(3 discs per serving – 170 calories)
DIET: GF

Now, just look here: these aren't the most elegant snack, oh no – but if you're looking for something nibbly, they won't steer you too wrong. Also, they're great for taking along to, oh, I don't know, nights of taste at certain slimming clubs. I say that, but if you're anything like us you'll package them up, eat them in the car park and then sack off the slimming club entirely because you'll have put on a pound of pure cheese.

Mind, we're not fans of those 'taster night' events: partly because I like to know how clean the kitchen that prepared my food is, partly because I don't like being pushed to the floor by Susan in her haste to force an extra wedge of soaking wet quiche into her gob, partly because I don't like the fact that the only drink offered is warm cherryade or Mellow Bird's coffee. It's a tough life: we settle for having a chippy tea on the way home to compromise.

2 bacon rashers, diced
4 tbsp passata
½ tsp garlic granules
¼ tsp dried mixed herbs
300g (10½oz) reduced-fat
    mozzarella cheese, grated
a handful of small fresh basil
    leaves

Preheat your grill to medium-high.

Spray a small frying pan or saucepan with a little oil and place over a medium-high heat. Add the diced bacon and quickly fry until starting to turn crispy around the edges.

Remove from the heat, add the passata, garlic granules and mixed herbs, and stir to warm through.

Line a baking tray with greaseproof paper or use a non-stick tray. Divide the cheese into about 12 neat piles and place on the tray (you might need to use two trays).

Place under the grill and cook until the mounds have melted into discs and browned, then remove from the heat.

Leave to cool for a few minutes, then top with a teaspoon or two of the passata mix.

Top each one with a small basil leaf.

SMART SWAPS

Mozzarella works best here, but you can also use Cheddar, or a blend if you prefer!

Swap the bacon for whatever you like – chorizo also works really well, as does a bit of shredded chicken.

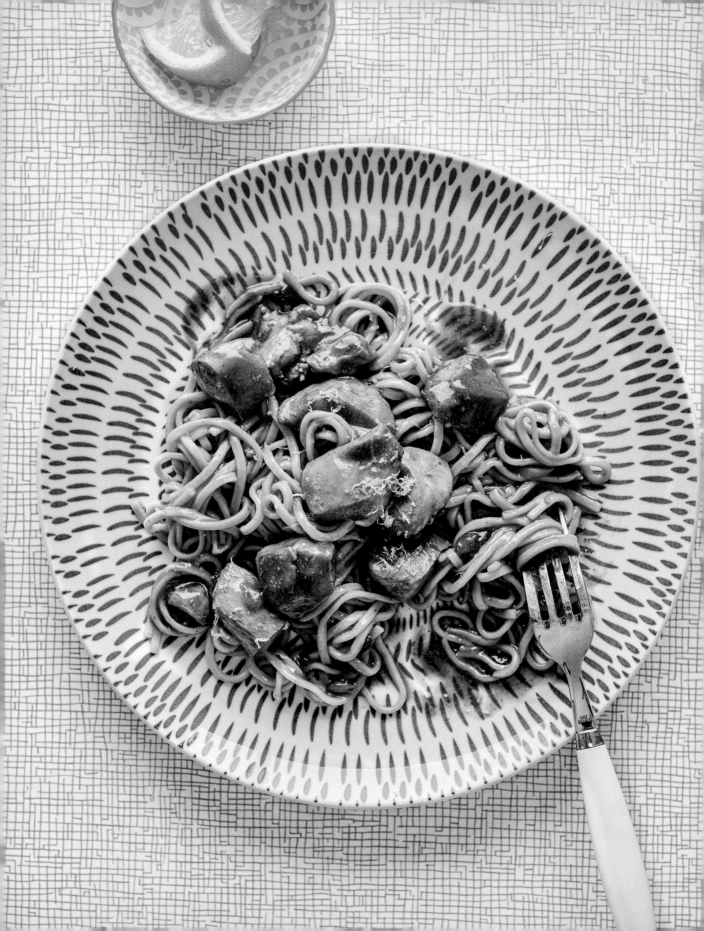

BEST-EVER LEMON CHICKEN FAKEAWAY

SERVES: 4
PREP: 5 minutes
(plus 1 hour marinating)
COOK: 20 minutes
CALORIES: 235

Lemon chicken is one of those dishes that people seem to feel ashamed about ordering from a takeaway: perhaps because it is super-simple, perhaps because it isn't the most exciting of meals – but balls to that, it's delicious. We spent a while trying to perfect the recipe for the blog and ended up over-complicating it, so here is our guaranteed gorgeousness in its most basic form. Enjoy!

Oh, and while totally unauthentic, you can absolutely swap out the lemon for orange.

Quick confession: the first time I had this was as a young'un while being babysat by one of my aunts. I enjoyed it terribly but my cousin took all the big chunks of chicken away from me because she was hungry/feral. I responded in kind by shutting her fingers in a door. Don't ever touch my food.

4 skinless, boneless chicken
    breasts, diced
3 tbsp light soy sauce
2 tbsp rice vinegar
175ml (6fl oz) chicken stock
75ml (2½fl oz) lemon juice
    (freshly squeezed is best)
2 tbsp honey
1 tbsp cornflour
zest of 1 lemon

Toss the chicken with the soy sauce and rice vinegar, then cover and leave to marinate in the fridge for an hour.

Heat a large frying pan over a medium-high heat. Add the chicken with its marinade and cook for 10–12 minutes, until cooked through.

Mix together the chicken stock, lemon juice, honey and cornflour. Add to the pan, stirring frequently, until thickened.

Sprinkle over the lemon zest and serve.

NOTE
Serve with rice or noodles
(or whatever you fancy!).

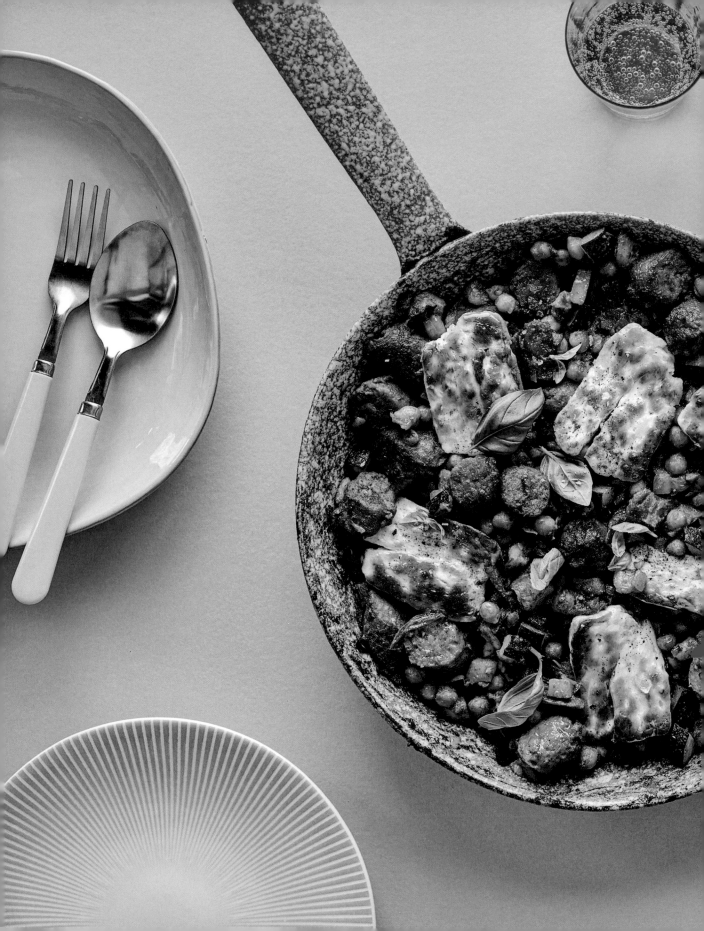

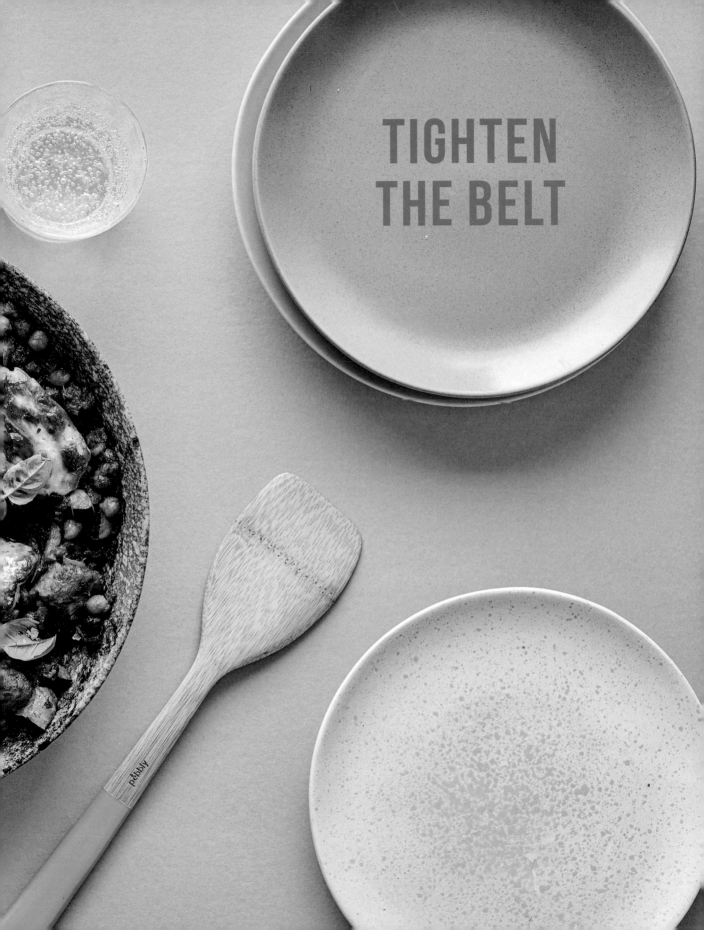

TIGHTEN
THE BELT

STEPS SALAD

SERVES: 2 as a main
or 4 as a starter
PREP: 5 minutes
COOK: 5 minutes
CALORIES: 176

The author of the emotional support potatoes from the previous book presents this salad for your consideration (positive feedback only). Ostensibly called Steps Salad because it has five steps, the real reason is because he wanted to shoehorn in a reference to his favourite band. Fair. I threatened to leave it out, but he said you'll be sorry – and he's a nightmare when he isn't happy: full stomp. No fear though, the tragedy of omitting such a delicious simple dinner from this book was the last thing on my mind.

This recipe serves two for a big substantial dinner, but also works as a lovely light starter for four if you share. Paul often asks me to make double and I say, I will, love, again.

Sigh.

a big handful of rocket leaves (or indeed, any 'fiery' green leaf)
1 large jar of roasted red peppers
100g (3½oz) reduced-fat halloumi
65g (2½oz) chorizo (cut into rings, or bought pre-chopped)
a few tablespoons of balsamic vinegar (the decent stuff)

Arrange the rocket in a pleasing manner on a plate.

Heat a small frying pan over a medium-high heat. Drain, dry and slice the roasted red peppers, warm them through in the frying pan, then place atop the rocket.

Slice the halloumi and brown on both sides in the frying pan, then add to the salad.

Add the chorizo to the pan and fry (without adding oil) until crispy, then add to the salad.

Add the balsamic to the chorizo and pepper oil in the pan and heat through, then drizzle over the salad.

NOTES

Occasionally served with hot spoons.

Feel free to make this 'fresher' by eschewing jarred peppers for fresh, but the smokiness of the jarred peppers adds a lot to the dish.

If you're not pushed for time, some cubed and roasted sweet potato or pumpkin will add an interesting texture experience.

No, I don't know what a texture experience is either, but I saw it on a menu once and thought it sounded right fancy, so go with it.

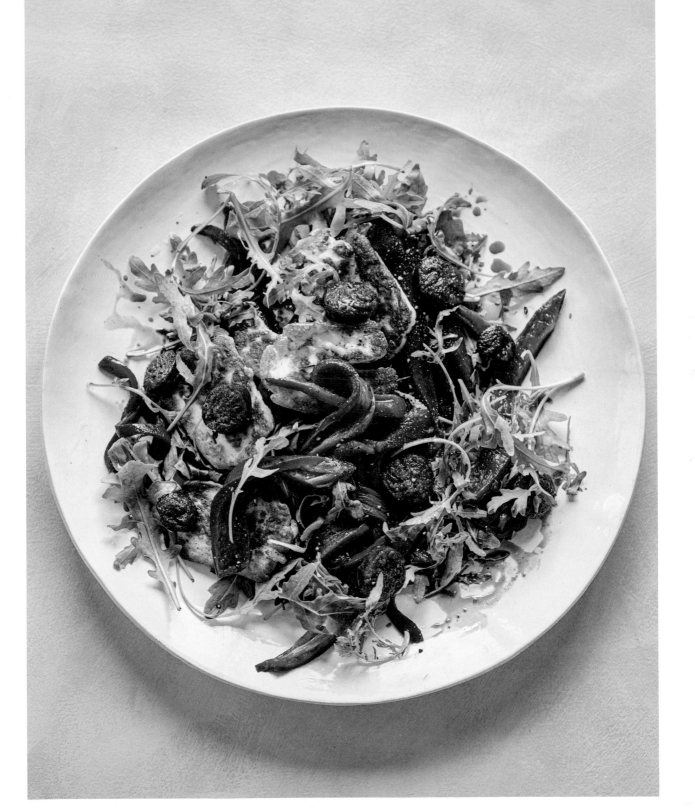

CHAFED (CHICKEN) THIGHS

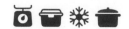

SERVES: 4
PREP: 10 minutes
COOK: 25 minutes
CALORIES: 248

We're calling these chafed thighs despite the fact they're clearly a little charred, but see, I wanted a reason to reference my thighs in the book. So indulgent, I know. Chafed thighs make me think of the one thing I've always wanted to crack but never quite got the hang of: running.

I have friends who run all day long (they're robbers, kaboom-tish) and can't stop telling me of the benefits, so, every now and then and mainly to get away from their smug faces, I'll try and start. I've downloaded all those apps that encourage you to run, but nothing seems to stick with me. I never get that 'rush' that people describe: I just get ankles that look like someone kicked them down a lift-shaft and a heaving chest. And look: I'm naturally buxom, I don't need them to heave as well.

I think I know why running doesn't work for me: I can't perfect that face that so many runners seem to have when they're running, where it looks as though they're both about to climax and itching to tell you about how good they feel. Maybe it's that, or the fact that so many parts of my body rub together when I move that adding speed into the friction renders everything sore and, well, chafed.

Anyway. Speaking of a sight for sore thighs …

2 tsp smoked paprika
2 tsp garlic granules
1 tsp onion granules
1 tsp black pepper
¼ tsp cayenne pepper
8 skinless, boneless chicken thighs
2 courgettes, quartered lengthways
4 cloves of garlic, crushed
juice of ½ lime
60ml (2fl oz) chicken stock
1 tsp dried chilli flakes

Mix together the paprika, garlic granules, onion granules, black pepper and cayenne pepper and rub into the chicken thighs.

Spray a large pan with a little oil and place it over a medium heat. Add the chicken and cook for 6–7 minutes each side, then remove from the heat and set aside.

Spray the pan with a little more oil and add the courgettes and crushed garlic. Cook for 4–5 minutes, gently stirring now and again.

Add the lime juice and stock, stir gently again, and cook for 3–4 minutes, stirring occasionally, until slightly reduced.

Put the chicken back into the pan and increase the heat to high. Cook for 2–3 minutes, then sprinkle over the chilli flakes and serve.

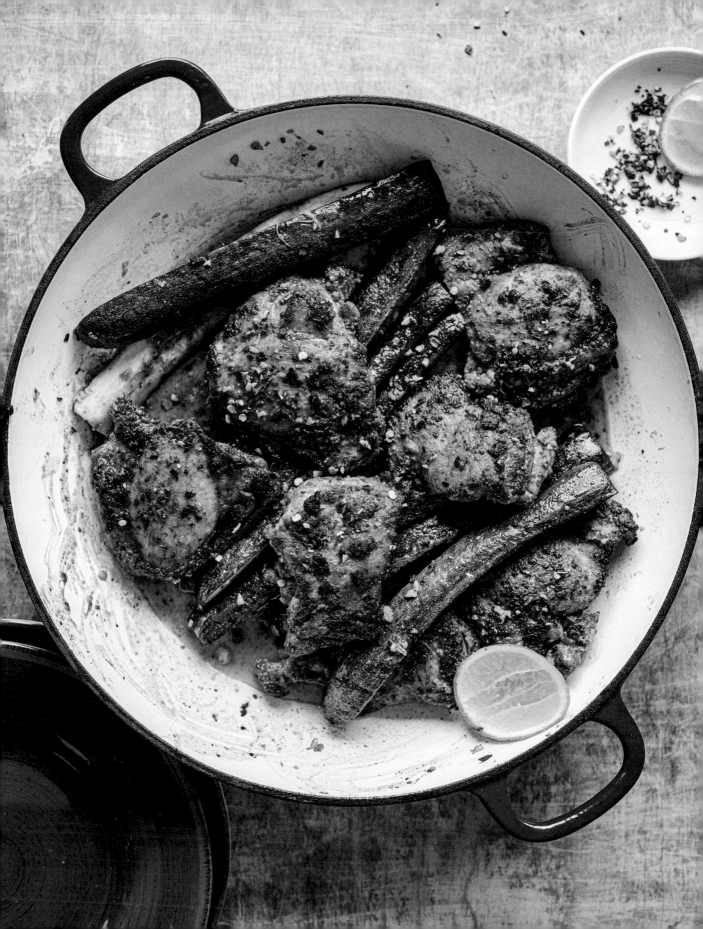

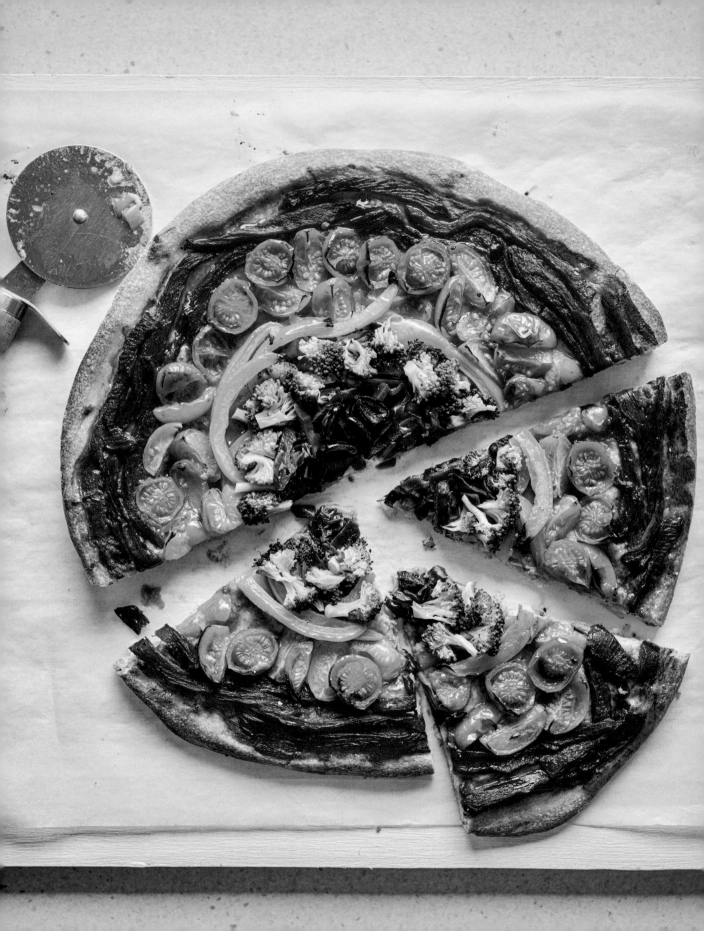

PRIDE PIZZA

SERVES: 2
PREP: 50 minutes
COOK: 15 minutes
CALORIES: 417
DIET: VEG/V/DF

This recipe from our blog was made for two reasons: we wanted something colourful to celebrate Pride month, and I wanted to get some vitamins into Paul. Curious how someone can rail against eating vegetables until they're on a pizza …

Pride is incredibly important to us. We're not shy about our sexuality, but that comes with the luxury of being two confident men who are built like brick shithouses. The world is not so golden for others out there, and that's why we make a big thing about it on the blog. We hope we may get to a point where sexuality is as irrelevant as 95% of the holes on Paul's belt, but it seems unlikely for a while.

But as long as we are kind, supportive and, most importantly, fabulous, perhaps we'll get there. To the pizza then. Can't be arsed making the dough? Chuck it on a pre-made base or even a wrap. We won't tell a soul.

For the dough
125g (4½oz) strong white bread flour
½ × 7g sachet of fast-action yeast
75ml (2½fl oz) warm water
1 tsp salt

For the pizza topping
150ml (5fl oz) passata
2 red peppers, chopped (see notes)
200g (7oz) orange cherry tomatoes, cut into quarters
1 yellow pepper, chopped
100g (3½oz) broccoli florets
75g (2¾oz) pickled red cabbage, chopped
8 pitted black olives, halved

Mix together the flour, yeast, warm water and salt in a bowl and knead until you get a ball of dough (or chuck it all into a mixer with a bread hook if you're a fanny like us).

Cover the bowl with clingfilm and leave in a warm place for about 30 minutes for it to rise.

Preheat the oven to 180°C fan/400°F/gas mark 6.

Roll or stretch the dough out to a pizza shape about 25–30cm (10–12 inches) across.

Spread the passata over the dough, right up to the edge.

Arrange your veg over the top, starting with the 'red' layer around the outside edge, and then repeating with the other 'colours'. Don't worry about being too neat.

Bake in the oven for about 15 minutes.

NOTES
For the 'red' ring, we like to use jarred roasted red peppers, just to add a bit more flavour!

SMART SWAP
The ingredients used here for the colours are a guide – obviously if you're not a fan, just swap them out for something you do like!

LEMON & HERB TURKEY KEBABS

SERVES: 4
PREP: 10 minutes
(plus 30 minutes marinating)
COOK: 15 minutes
CALORIES: 164
DIET: GF/DF

4 skinless, boneless turkey
   breasts, cubed
4 tbsp lemon juice
3 cloves of garlic, crushed
1 tsp dried thyme
2 tsp dried rosemary
1 tsp dried mixed herbs
1 tsp salt
1 tsp black pepper

These turkey kebabs will fill your soul with sunshine, we promise, and the recipe below is perfect for a quick dinner served over salad or folded into a wrap. While you have the thyme, garlic and lemon juice to hand, you could boost this dinner further by making a bowl of lemon and garlic roast potatoes.

No exact science: just dice up some new potatoes, coat them in lemon juice and olive oil, lots of crushed garlic and add a pinch of salt, thyme and pepper. Roast in the oven while you prepare the turkey kebabs and there you have it, a whole dinner of magic.

How's that for efficiency, though: a hidden recipe in the intro! We do spoil you lot.

If you're using wooden skewers, make sure to soak them for a good 30 minutes beforehand, so they don't burn.

Pop the turkey into a large bowl, add the lemon juice, garlic, thyme, rosemary, mixed herbs, salt and black pepper, and give it all a good toss.

Cover with clingfilm and leave to marinate for 30 minutes.

Carefully thread the turkey onto the skewers (one per serving, so four in total).

Preheat the grill to medium-high and cook the turkey for 15 minutes, turning every few minutes.

Serve!

NOTE
These also work great on a barbecue!

SMART SWAPS
Use any herbs you like on these, whatever you have in your cupboards – slap 'em on!

If you can't get hold of turkey, chicken works just as well.

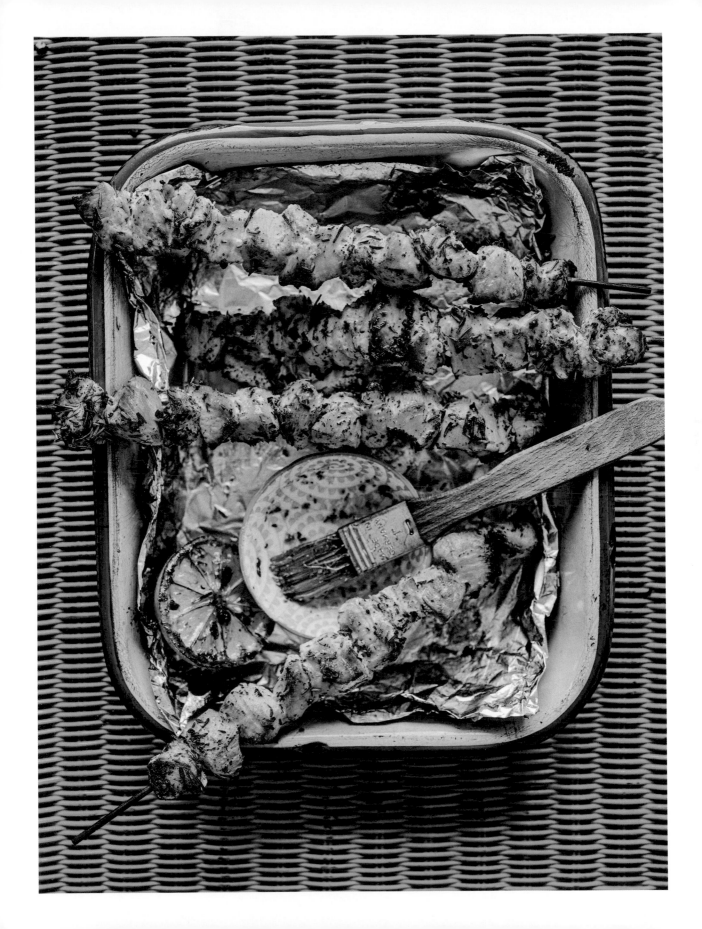

OUR BEST-EVER CHOW MEIN

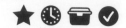

SERVES: 4
PREP: 10 minutes
(plus a few hours marinating)
COOK: 10 minutes
CALORIES: 425
DIET: DF

1 tsp cornflour
2 tbsp dark soy sauce
4 tbsp light soy sauce
5 tbsp oyster sauce
100g (3½oz) of whatever cooked meat you have (we've used beef)
2–3 dried noodle nests
1 large onion, chopped
2 cloves of garlic, crushed
1 tsp black pepper
5 spring onions, sliced thinly
1 large red pepper, sliced thinly
350g (12oz) beansprouts
1 tsp granulated sugar
1 tbsp sesame oil

That's a big old list of ingredients there, but you need to hear me out: you'll have most of this in your cupboards, and whatever you haven't got, just substitute with something else. Be sensible: don't be swapping oyster sauce for beef gravy or that bottle of bleach you stir into your mother-in-law's tea. Just me? OK.

This recipe is an absolute joy because it really does taste exactly like one you would order from a takeaway: it also lends itself to whatever leftover meat and vegetables you may have sitting around in the fridge. As we say to all the married men we meet, you mustn't be afraid to experiment.

Mix the cornflour with 1 tablespoon of dark soy sauce, 1 tablespoon of light soy sauce and 2 tablespoons of oyster sauce. Pour this over the meat and leave to marinate for a few hours.

Cook the noodles according to the packet instructions, then drain and rinse under cold water.

Heat a large saucepan or wok over a medium-high heat and spray it with a little oil.

Add the meat with its marinade and cook for a few minutes until warmed through, then remove to a plate.

Spray the pan with a bit more oil and turn the heat to high, then add the onion, garlic, black pepper, spring onions, red pepper and beansprouts and cook quickly but thoroughly for a few minutes.

Put the meat back into the pan along with the rest of the soy sauces and oyster sauce, drained noodles, sugar and sesame oil, and stir continuously until everything is warmed through.

Serve!

SMART SWAP

Adjust the quantity of meat to whatever you like, it really doesn't matter – you can use anything: pork, chicken, beef, duck ... This is GREAT for using up the scraps from a roast dinner. Or, don't have any meat at all!

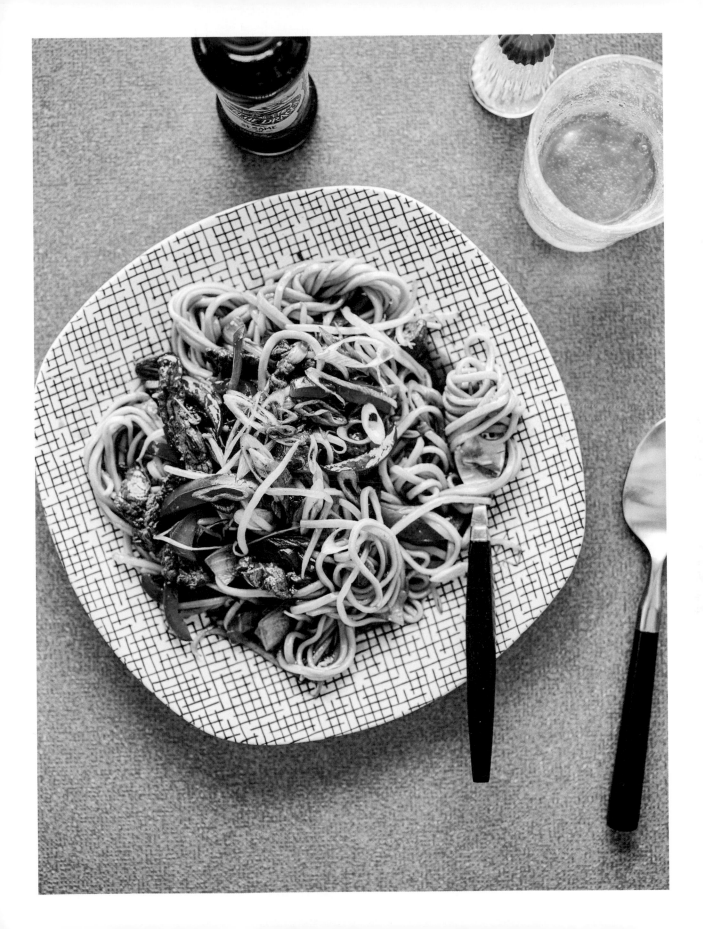

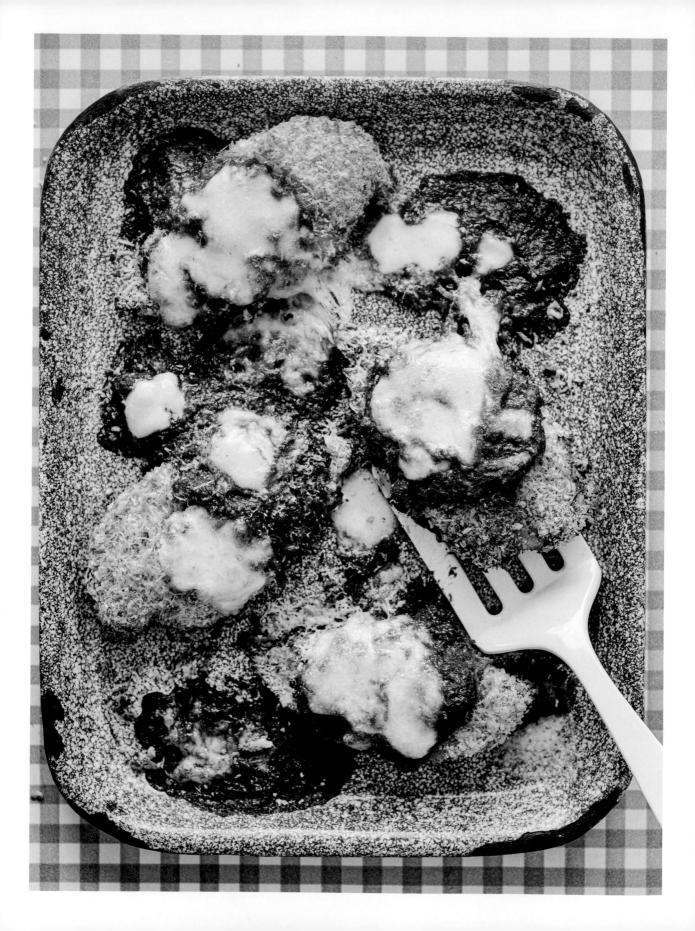

CHUBBY CHICKEN PARMO

SERVES: 4
PREP: 5 minutes
COOK: 25 minutes
CALORIES: 347

Let me correct one thing almost immediately: when I last referenced a parmo as a Geordie delicacy (never again), I received such a torrent of abuse and correction from the fine people of Middlesbrough that I feared for my kneecaps. Not because they're a violent sort, mind, simply because we had so many invitations to try their parmos that my legs were pulling out from under me in their independent haste to take the offers up.

A parmo is a terrific thing: as simple as butterflied chicken, with a tomato sauce and cheese strewn on the top until you have an ooey-gooey-wonder. There truly is no better food for the end of a heavy drinking session where you crave everything your mother warned you about. Get it in you!

4 skinless, boneless chicken breasts
2 eggs, beaten
70g (2½oz) panko breadcrumbs
1 × 400g (14oz) tin of peeled plum tomatoes
4 cloves of garlic
½ onion, finely diced
¼ tsp dried oregano
½ tsp onion powder
100g (3½oz) reduced-fat mozzarella cheese, grated
25g (1oz) Parmesan cheese, grated

Preheat the oven to 200°C fan/425°F/gas mark 7.

Wrap each chicken breast in clingfilm and give it a good whack with a rolling pin (or whatever you have to hand) until it's about 2.5cm (1 inch) thick.

One at a time, dip the chicken breasts into the beaten egg, then slap them on to a plate of breadcrumbs, making sure they are well coated.

Gently place the chicken breasts on a baking sheet and bake in the oven for about 15 minutes.

Meanwhile, pop the tomatoes, garlic, onion, oregano and onion powder into a saucepan over a medium heat and bring to a simmer, stirring frequently.

Using a masher or a fork, break up the tomatoes as much as you can to make a pulpy sauce (see note).

Keep simmering for another 10 minutes or so.

Remove the chicken from the oven, pour over the tomato sauce, and top with the grated cheese. Put back into the oven for another 5–10 minutes.

Serve!

NOTE

If you want a smooth sauce, blend it with a stick blender, but honestly, it's fine lumpy.

TIGHTEN THE BELT

CRACKING LAMB BALLS

SERVES: 4
PREP: 15 minutes
COOK: 25 minutes
CALORIES: 307
DIET: GF/DF

One of the surprise hits from the previous book was our lamb and halloumi meatballs, which people filled our social media streams with. We were pleased indeed because in all honesty we thought the sight of them – big balls with lumps of cheese sticking out – were so ungainly that it would put people off. We should have known better!

So Paul is doubling down on the success and, in the interest of being smutty, has created these lamb balls – and quite honestly, they're delicious. They remind me of those little frikadellen balls you can buy in petrol stations, and that's no bad thing: as someone who spends a lot of time travelling, I have extensively reviewed the various ranges on offer. If you need someone to walk you through the finer points of motorway cuisine, do give me a shout.

Curiously, for someone who doesn't drive a lorry, I also know my way around most of the UK's lorry parks …

1 onion, finely diced
3 cloves of garlic, crushed
2 tsp ground cumin
1 tsp ground coriander
1 tsp dried chilli flakes
1 × 400g (14oz) tin of chickpeas, drained
400g (14oz) lamb mince
2 tsp mint sauce

Heat a small frying pan over a medium heat and spray it with a little oil.

Add the onion and cook for 3–4 minutes.

Add the garlic, cumin, coriander and chilli flakes and cook for another 2 minutes, then remove from the heat and set aside to cool.

Pop the chickpeas into a food processor and blitz until smooth.

In a bowl, mix together the chickpeas, cooked onion mix, lamb mince and mint sauce.

Spoon out about a tablespoon of the mixture at a time and roll it into balls. Repeat until you've used all the mixture.

Spray a large frying pan with a little oil and place it over a medium heat. Add the balls to the pan and cook until brown and cooked through, about 10–15 minutes.

Serve.

NOTES

These go great with some some tzatziki (see page 146) or houmous.

Serve with rice or flatbreads (use gluten-free ones if that's your dietary requirement).

TIGHTEN THE BELT

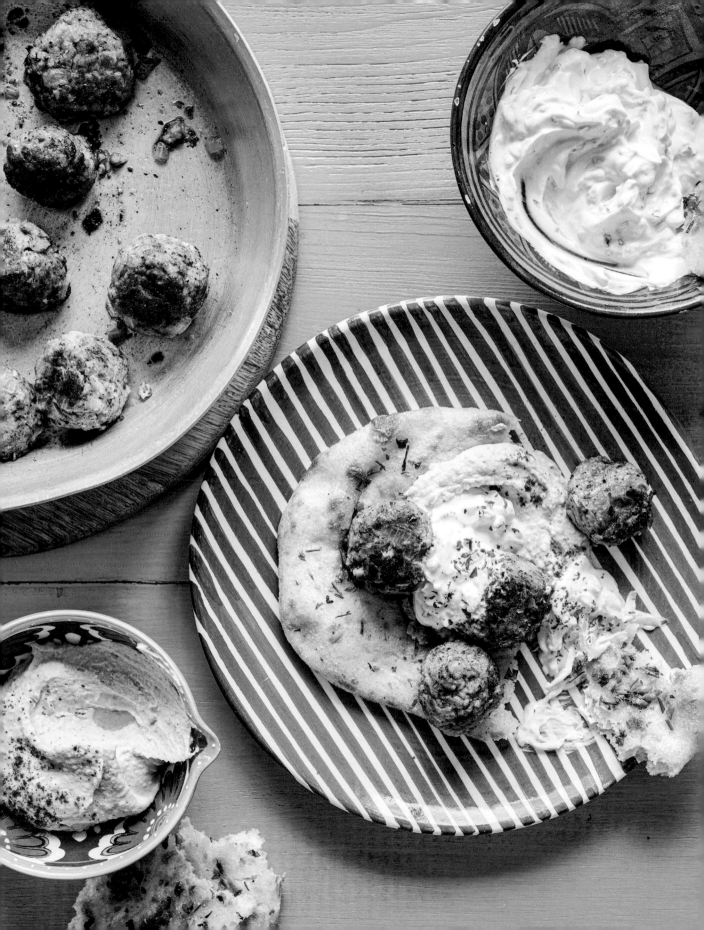

MEDITERRANEAN HALLOUMI TRAYBAKE

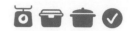

SERVES: 4
PREP: 10 minutes
COOK: 45 minutes
CALORIES: 418
DIET: VEG (check halloumi is vegetarian friendly)

In the last book I made a rash promise to Paul: he could get a dog if the book sold well. Unfortunately, it did, and I had to explain to him that sometimes what I say and what I do are entirely different things.

You must understand: I'd bloody love a dog. My teenage years were spent walking our collie Oscar, who was scared of loud noises. The summer they brought bird-bangers (machines that emulate a shotgun bang to scare birds away) into the fields near me, I'd walk Oscar into arse-end nowhere only for them to start and for him to go barrelling off across the fields. I lost three stone that summer just chasing him.

He was happy and died at an old age in his sleep. But, as a result, I can't cope with the inevitable end of any potential dog, so it's off the cards. Sorry, Paul.

Why am I mentioning this here? It's bloody hard to make an interesting intro about a halloumi bake. Forgive me.

8 vegetarian sausages
1 onion, diced
2 courgettes, diced
4 tomatoes, diced
1 tsp salt
1 tbsp ground turmeric
1 tbsp ground cumin
1 tsp cayenne pepper
1 × 400g (14oz) tin of chickpeas, drained
200g (7oz) halloumi cheese, sliced
1 tbsp chopped fresh basil

Heat the grill to medium-high.

Brown the sausages under the grill, turning regularly, then set aside to cool and slice (don't worry if they're not cooked all the way through).

Heat an ovenproof pan over a medium-high heat and spray it with a little oil.

Add the onion to the pan and cook for a few minutes, then add the sliced sausages and cook for a few minutes more.

Add the courgettes and tomatoes to the pan, along with the salt, turmeric, cumin, cayenne pepper and chickpeas.

Simmer over a medium-high heat for 20 minutes. Meanwhile heat the grill to medium-high again.

Lay the sliced halloumi on top of the mix and place under the grill for a few minutes until golden.

Sprinkle with the chopped basil and serve.

SMART SWAP

If you're partial to a meatier sausage, pork ones work well instead of veggie ones.

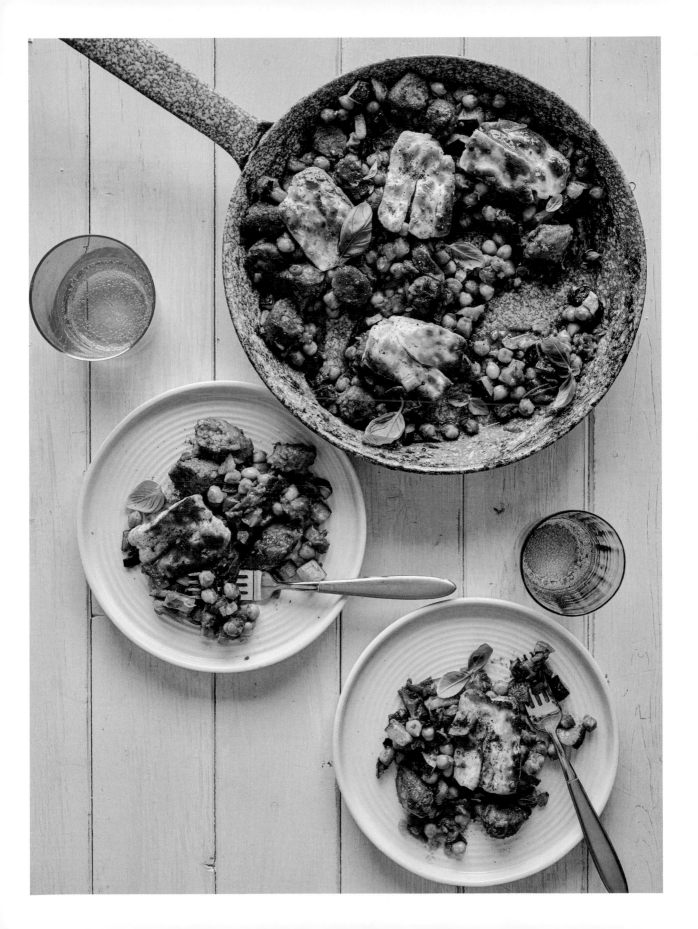

SWEET & SOUR CHICKEN MEATBALLS

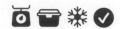

SERVES: 4
PREP: 20 minutes
COOK: 20 minutes
CALORIES: 265
DIET: DF

All right, so it's my turn. You heard all about how wonderful I am, back at the poutine. Know that I was very much guilt-tripped into writing this, being given a sharp deadline as James fired the Citroën up the hill to get some more Tangfastics from Morrisons.

I thought this was the perfect recipe to showcase all my muffin, James, means to me – he's both sweet and sour. Let me explain.

Sweet? Absolutely. I've lost count of all the thoughtful things he's done for me out of the blue, from big gestures such as surprise holidays to New York, or little things like squirting out a heart in smooth pickle on my sandwiches. Admittedly, they mostly make an appearance when he's after something/binned something important, but they're still lovely nonetheless. Sour? There's nowt we love more than a good bedtime bitch sesh. We're like a pair of cackling hags, calling each and every person we know. And we love it.

Right, recipe.

For the meatballs
500g (1lb 2oz) chicken mince
30g (1oz) panko breadcrumbs
4 spring onions, finely chopped,
    plus extra for ganish
3 cloves of garlic, crushed
5cm (2 inches) ginger, grated
1 tsp sesame oil
1 tbsp light or dark soy sauce

For the sauce
2 tsp cornflour
80ml (2¾fl oz) light or dark
    soy sauce
1 tbsp cider vinegar
1 clove of garlic, crushed
3 tbsp honey
1 tsp sesame oil

Preheat the oven to 220°C fan/475°F/gas mark 9.

In a bowl, mix together all the meatball ingredients.

Divide the mixture into about 24 meatballs and roll them into shape, then place them on a baking sheet lined with greaseproof paper and bake in the oven for 15–20 minutes.

Meanwhile, mix the cornflour with 2 teaspoons of water. Mix with the rest of the sauce ingredients and pour into a small saucepan. Gently bring to the boil, then reduce to a simmer, whisking frequently.

When the meatballs are cooked, remove them from the oven and drizzle over the sauce, rolling them around to ensure they're well coated.

Sprinkle with spring onions and serve.

NOTES
If you prefer a runnier sauce, leave out the cornflour.

Serve with rice.

SMART SWAP
Turkey, pork and even beef mince are great in this!

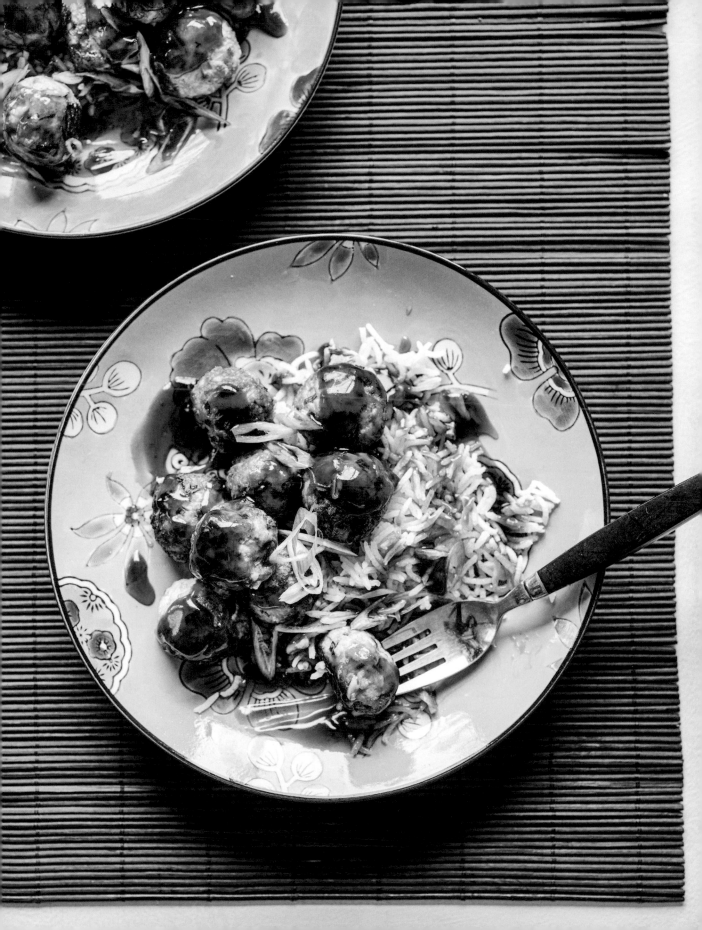

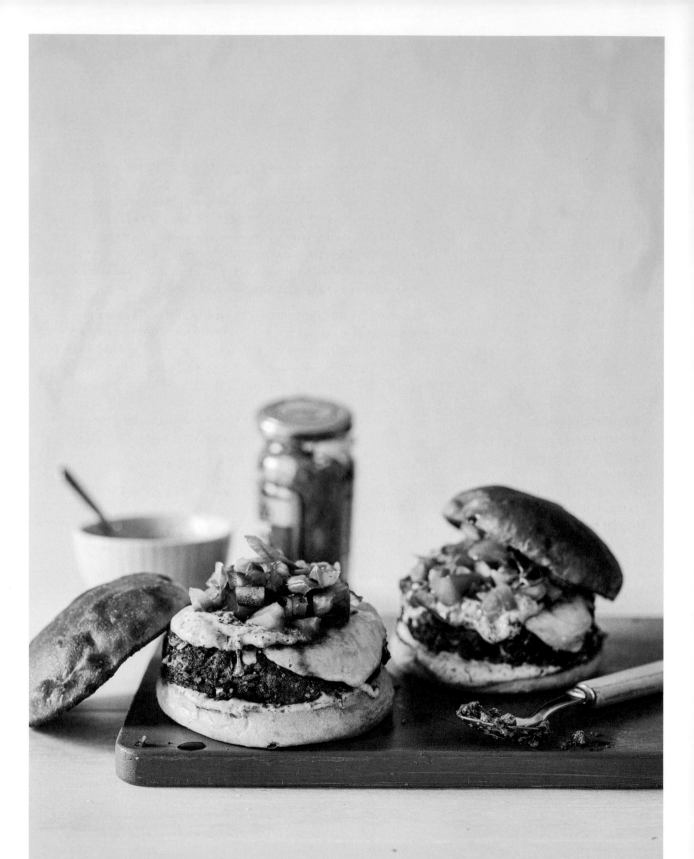

PESTO QUORN BURGERS

SERVES: 4
PREP: 20 minutes
COOK: 10 minutes
CALORIES: 399
DIET: VEG (check pesto and mozzarella are vegetarian friendly)

Quite a long recipe here, so I'm going to do you a favour and keep my ramblings short. It doesn't come naturally to me because goodness me does writing a blog give you an ability for spinning a story. I rage as much as you do when I click on to a blog to try and get a recipe for soup only to have to wade through 2,500 words about Alice's Adventures in Mediocrity, but look, forgive me: I've always wanted to be a writer and this is my only outlet. I do try to slip in as many knob-jokes as I can to keep you going, mind – because I care.

These pesto burgers, though: they're utterly terrific. If you were feeling especially outrageous, you could use sun-dried tomato pesto instead of the basil variety: it is wonderful. Though I'll say this, if your idea of being outrageous is swapping out your condiments, then we really need to have a word. Enjoy!

40g (1½oz) couscous
4 tbsp extra-light mayonnaise
5 tsp reduced-fat pesto
250g (9oz) Quorn mince
2 spring onions, sliced
¼ tsp garlic granules
60g (2¼oz) mozzarella cheese, grated
4 buns
2 tomatoes, chopped
a handful of fresh basil leaves, finely chopped
2 tsp balsamic vinegar

Place the couscous in a heatproof bowl and pour over boiling water until just covered, then put a plate on top and leave for 5–10 minutes.

Mix the mayonnaise with 1 teaspoon of the pesto and set aside.

In a bowl, mix together the Quorn mince, couscous, spring onions, garlic granules and the remaining pesto.

Divide the mixture into four balls and squash them down to make burger shapes.

Heat a large frying pan over a medium-high heat and spray it with a little oil. Cook the burgers for 4–5 minutes each side, topping with the mozzarella for the last couple of minutes.

As the burgers are cooking, slice and gently toast the buns either under a hot grill or in a toaster.

Spread the bottom halves of the buns with pesto mayonnaise, place the burgers on top, top with the chopped tomato and basil, and drizzle with the balsamic vinegar. Add the top half of each bun and serve!

NOTE

People often add an egg to a burger mixture but it really isn't necessary.

SMART SWAP

You can swap out the Quorn mince for chicken mince if you fancy a meatier mouthful.

TIGHTEN THE BELT

NICELY SPICY EASY CHEESY YELLOW BUTTERNUT LINGUINE

SERVES: 4
PREP: 15 minutes
COOK: 30 minutes
CALORIES: 492

Normally I would apologize for such a gloriously laboured pun, but you know what – I'll own it. The way our recipe development works is that Paul will toil endlessly in the kitchen, coming up with new ideas, spins on recipes we have done before and tasty alternatives. My input at this stage is minimal and consists of nothing more than trying the food, giving him a wan smile if it's delicious and hurling the pan and contents across the kitchen if it isn't up to scratch. I joke, of course: I'm neither that fiery in temper or insouciant regarding food waste.

However, occasionally I'll have an amazing idea, and so when Paul laughed his brittle, fractured giggle, I knew this pun was a winner. The recipe below came *after* we agreed the title, and I genuinely believe it's one of the best.

1 red onion, chopped
2 cloves of garlic, crushed
600g (1lb 5oz) butternut squash, cut into 2cm (¾ inch) cubes
250ml (9fl oz) chicken stock
1½ tsp paprika
250g (9oz) linguine
200ml (7fl oz) milk
100g (3½oz) hot and spicy cheese (we use Mexicana brand), grated
4 bacon medallions, chopped
2 tsp sriracha
½ tsp dried chilli flakes

Spray a large saucepan with oil and place it over a medium heat. Add the onion and cook for about 2–3 minutes, then add the garlic and cook for another 30 seconds, stirring constantly.

Add the butternut squash to the pan, along with the chicken stock and paprika. Stir well, cover, and simmer for 15 minutes.

Meanwhile, bring a large pan of water to the boil. Cook the linguine according to the packet instructions, then drain, reserving half a mug of the cooking water.

When the squash has softened, remove the pan from the heat and stir in the milk. Blend with a stick blender until smooth, add the grated cheese, then place back over a medium heat to warm through, stirring occasionally.

Spray a frying pan with a little oil, place over a high heat and add the bacon. Cook until crispy, then remove from the heat and set aside.

Add the cooked and drained linguine to the pan of sauce and mix together. If it looks a little dry or stiff, add a few tablespoons of the reserved cooking water, a little at a time, until it's smooth again.

Serve, topped with the crispy bacon, a drizzle of sriracha and a sprinkle of chilli flakes.

SMART SWAP

You can adapt this to your liking by adding or reducing the chilli flakes and sriracha. It also works really well by replacing the sriracha with barbecue sauce if you like it a bit smokier and less spicy.

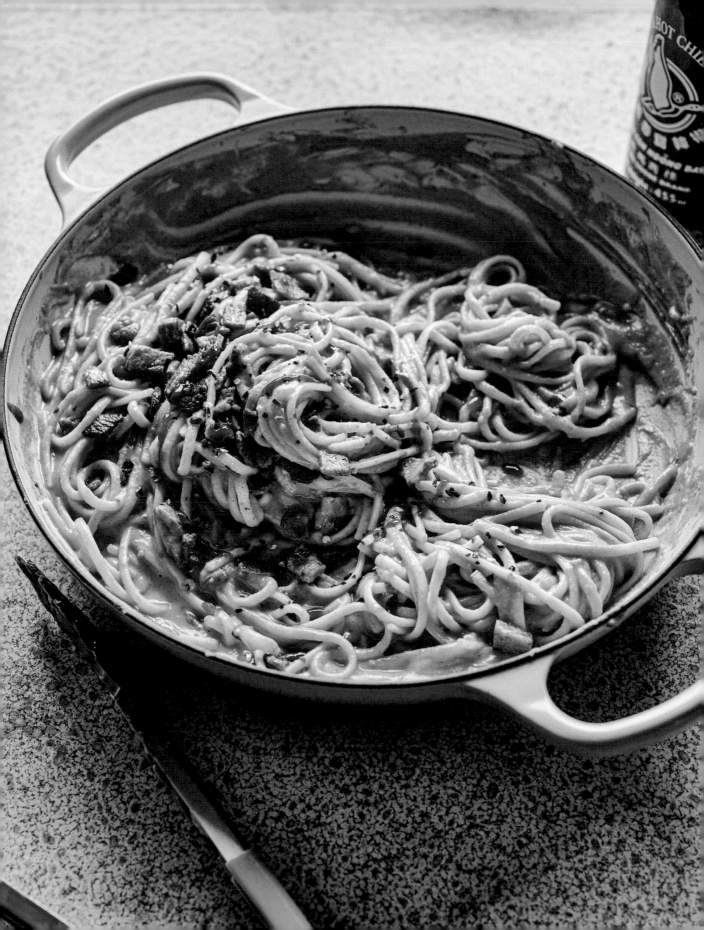

INDIAN SALAD

SERVES: 4
PREP: 20 minutes
COOK: 25 minutes
CALORIES: 326
DIET: DF/GF

We go through spells of salad at Chubby Towers: periods when we decide that everything we eat must come nicely diced and full of vitamins. That's why we have so many fresh takes on the simple salad, and this Indian-inspired wonder is definitely one of those.

If you're a delivery driver, you can probably work out when these spells hit by how many bags of clothes you're delivering to our house – I'll lose 4lb and decide I need a whole new wardrobe. What actually happens is that I'll try on everything I buy, then guiltily (and I am not someone to whom guilt comes easily) package it up and throw it into the boot of my car. There seems to be a mental barrier in my head when it comes to free returns: I can do the parcelling up, I can get them into the car, but going into the Post Office and handing everything over seems to be beyond the wit of man.

Though it's reassuring to know that if this twochubbycubs thing goes under, I can operate a satellite warehouse of gaudy 3XL T-shirts from my little Citroën. Always thinking ahead …

1 tsp ground turmeric
1 tsp dried mixed herbs
1 tsp dried thyme
1 tsp garlic granules
3 tbsp lemon juice
8 skinless, boneless chicken thighs
3 tbsp orange juice
½ tsp salt
1 tsp oil
2 romaine hearts, chopped
½ cucumber, diced
1 avocado, diced
¼ mango, diced
1 orange, peeled and cut into segments

Preheat the oven to 200°C/425°F/gas mark 7.

Mix together the turmeric, herbs, garlic granules and 2 tablespoons of lemon juice and rub into the chicken thighs.

Place the chicken on a baking sheet and cook in the oven for 15 minutes, then turn and cook for about 10 minutes.

Remove from the oven and allow to cool.

Meanwhile, mix together the remaining lemon juice, orange juice, salt and oil to make the dressing.

Assemble the salad by plating the lettuce, cucumber, avocado, mango and orange segments.

Roughly chop the chicken and divide among the plates.

Drizzle with the dressing and serve.

SMART SWAP

You can use chicken breasts if you prefer (but please do give thighs a go, they're so much nicer!) – just cook them in the oven for a few minutes longer each side.

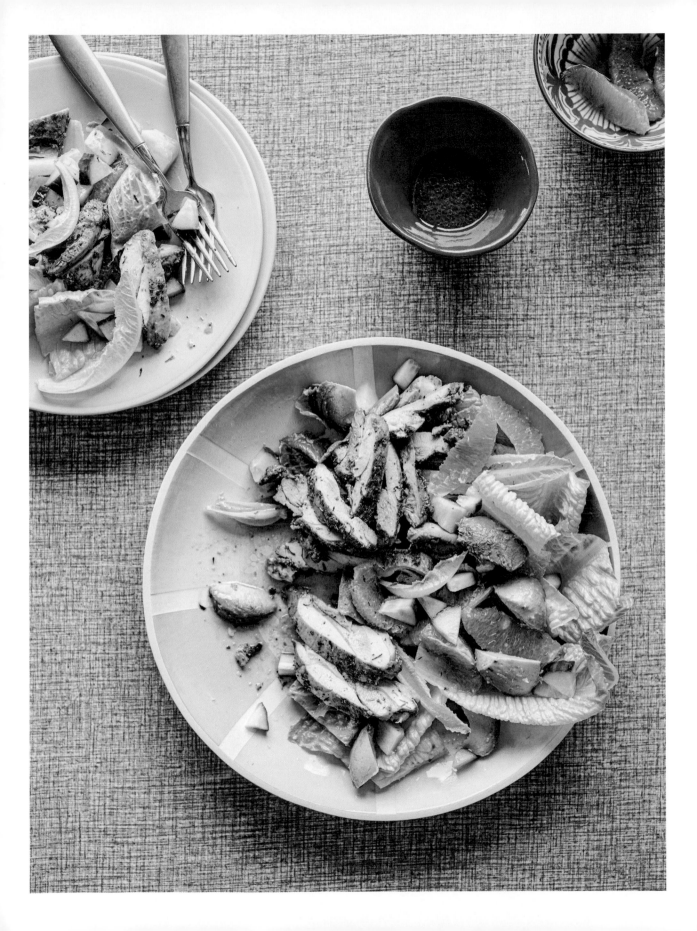

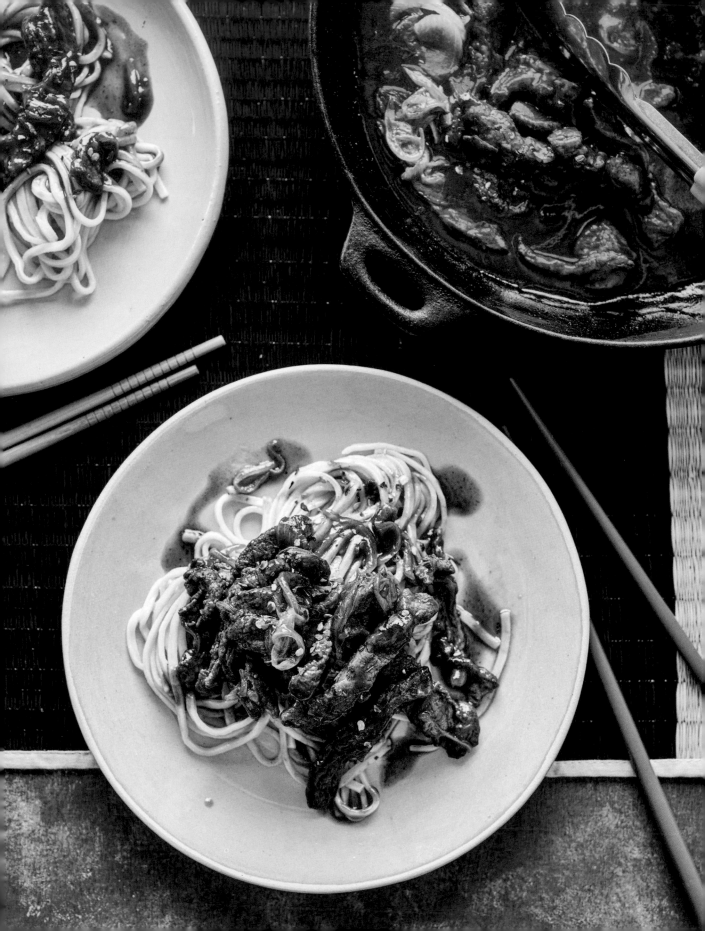

BEEF IN OK SAUCE

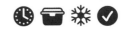

SERVES: 4
PREP: 10 minutes
COOK: 20 minutes
CALORIES: 274
DIET: DF

Beef in OK sauce doesn't sound very flash, does it? But trust us, for when have we ever steered you badly? OK sauce is like a fruitier brown sauce, and in the interests of being fast and filling we have made it from a couple of basic ingredients here. You're welcome to dig out a full recipe and we heartily encourage you to do so if you have the time.

If you are desperate to watch your calories, you can drop this still further by swapping the tomato sauce for passata and simmering it for a little longer until it thickens. But for quick and easy, this isn't terrible for your waistline.

If you were wanting to bulk the dish out, a couple of sliced peppers, an oriental mushroom mix and some baby corn really fills it out.

2 tsp light soy sauce
1 tsp Chinese five spice
120ml (4fl oz) tomato ketchup
4 tbsp brown sauce
3 tbsp brown sugar
cooking oil
1 onion, finely sliced
350g (12oz) stir-fry beef strips
a pinch of dried chilli flakes

Put the soy sauce, five spice, tomato ketchup, brown sauce and sugar into a saucepan along with 250ml (9fl oz) of water and gently bring to the boil, stirring continuously.

Reduce the heat and simmer for a few minutes, then remove from the heat and set aside.

Spray a large frying pan with oil and place over a medium-high heat.

Add the onion to the pan and fry for 2–3 minutes, stirring frequently.

Add the beef and stir for a few minutes until browned.

Finally, pour the sauce into the pan and stir to combine.

Sprinkle over the chilli flakes and serve.

NOTE

Serve with rice or noodles.

SMART SWAPS

Any meat will do for this, or even tofu if you're that way inclined. Just make sure that if you use meat it's cooked through properly.

White sugar can be used in place of brown, or you can swap some out for sweetener if you like.

TIGHTEN THE BELT

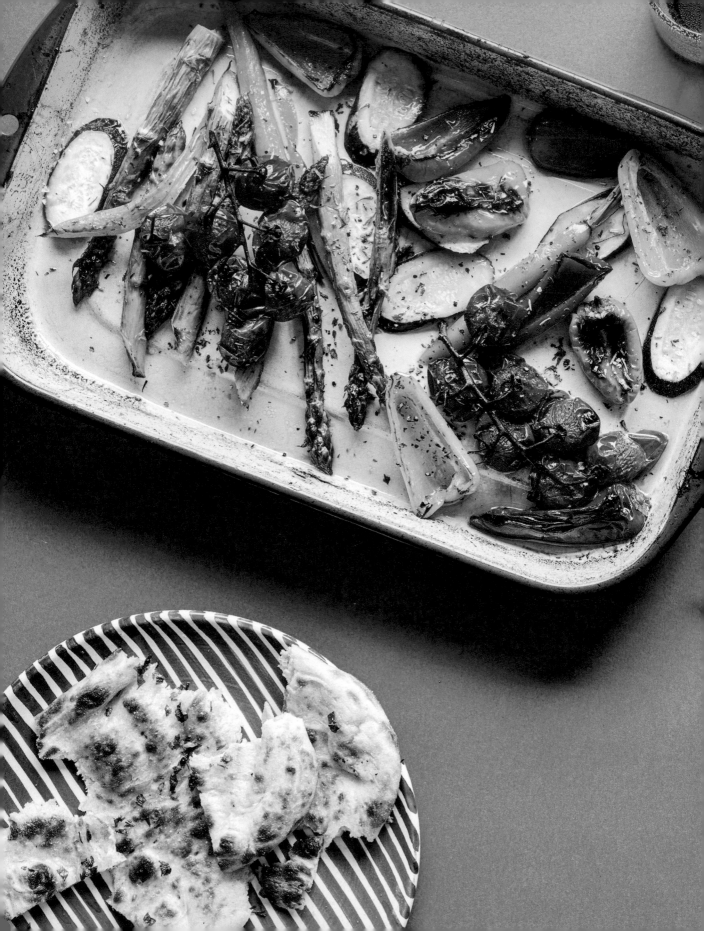

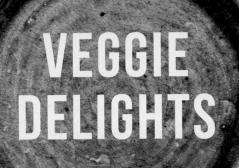

VEGGIE
DELIGHTS

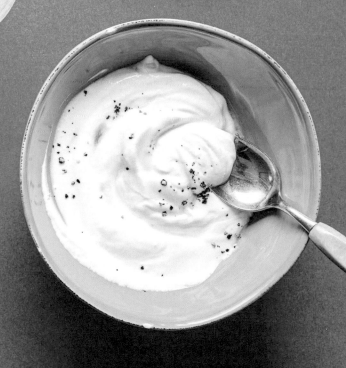

ROASTED CAULIFLOWER NUGGETS

SERVES: 4
PREP: 10 minutes
COOK: 40 minutes
CALORIES: 185
DIET: V/DF

Never before has a recipe left me shooketh quite as much as this one: it sounds like you're going to be eating a mouthful of fart, but actually, these are damn fine. The brother to the broccoli bombs from our blog, and one that I heartily encourage you to try. If you're feeling decadent, add some strong sharp cheese into the mixture. Sidenote: we've been trying to find a decent vegan cheese for a while now as we up our vegan recipe game on the blog, and are yet to crack it – if you can recommend a decent fauxmage, please do let us know.

Oh, come here a minute so I can whisper in your ear, will you? Don't tell a soul, but if you deep-fry them, they're even more incredible. But don't you be doing that, because this is a slimming book and such things must be discouraged. Honestly, have you no shame?

½ cauliflower, chopped into florets
25g (1oz) panko breadcrumbs
3 tbsp cornflour
2 tsp smoked paprika
1 tsp hot chilli powder
½ tsp garlic granules
½ tsp onion granules
½ tsp salt
1 tbsp nutritional yeast flakes
3 tbsp olive oil

Preheat the oven to 180°C fan/400°F/gas mark 6 and line a baking sheet with greaseproof paper.

Toss the cauliflower with all the other ingredients in a large bowl until well coated. Tip out on to a baking sheet and spread out into a single layer.

Bake in the oven for 20 minutes, then turn and cook for another 20 minutes.

Serve.

NOTES

Nutritional yeast is great stuff – you'll find it in most natural food or health shops. It gives a great nutty and cheesy flavour to things. If you haven't tried it yet, do – you'll love it.

This is a great way to get kids to eat vegetables – they'll love the flavour!

Have these as a main with some veg or salad, or as a side dish served with mayonnaise, or even as a snack!

If you don't like things too hot, you can leave out the chilli powder.

SMART SWAP

If you struggle to find panko breadcrumbs, ordinary breadcrumbs will do.

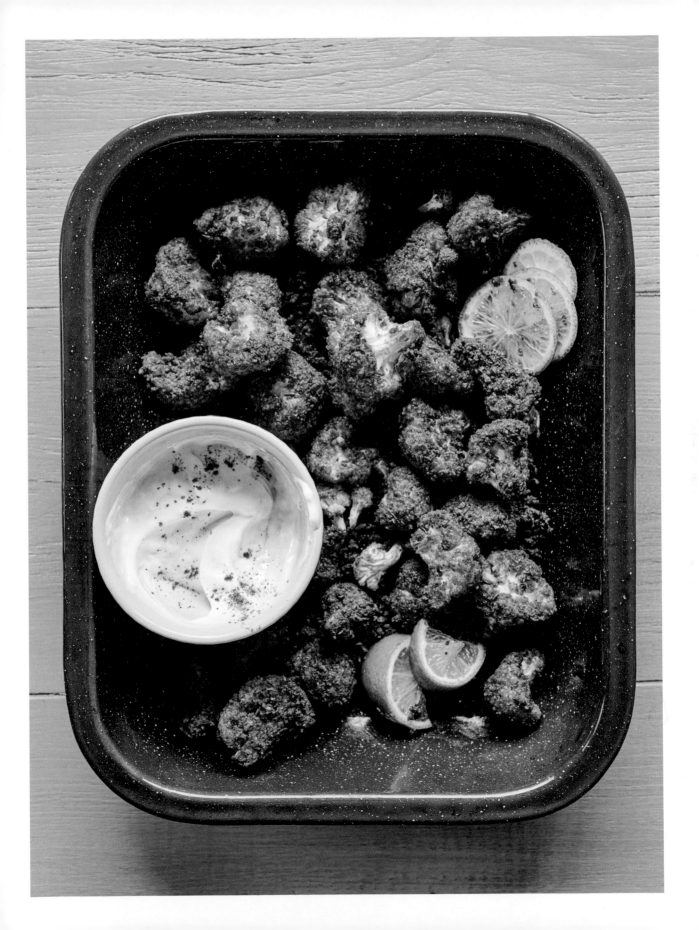

CACIO E PEPE

SERVES: 4
PREP: 5 minutes
COOK: 12 minutes
CALORIES: 497
DIET: VEG

Sometimes the best recipes are the simplest: there's a lot to be said for a meal that is on the table in minutes and uses only a few ingredients.

I say that – I can send Hurricane Paul into the kitchen to put some dry cat food down only to return to what looks like he's hurled a hand grenade in through the window. He has an incredible propensity for inexplicably using every single item we have in the kitchen, whether the recipe calls for it or not. By way of example, in making this recipe, he dug out our bulky food processor (I was foaming: I'd been using it to keep our loose nuts and bolts in) to grate the Parmesan rather than using the microplane grater.

He claimed his wrists were aching, which I can sympathize with: we've been married thirteen years at this point and there's a lot of DIY involved. But still.

Anyway, hush, James. Don't let them peek behind the curtain. This recipe can be bolstered with the addition of bacon or anchovies, but honestly, let the simplicity sing.

400g (14oz) spaghetti
125g (4½oz) vegetarian Italian
   hard cheese, grated
cracked black pepper
a pinch of salt

Cook the spaghetti according to the packet instructions, then drain (reserve half a mug of the cooking water).

Place a large frying pan over a medium-high heat and add the drained spaghetti to it.

Add about 6 tablespoons of the reserved pasta cooking water and give it a good toss.

Remove from the heat, add the grated cheese, and give it one good stir.

Leave it for a minute, then stir again and crack over the black pepper and salt.

Serve.

NOTE

The thing with the water seems like a faff, but it's worth doing – it stops the pasta getting too dry.

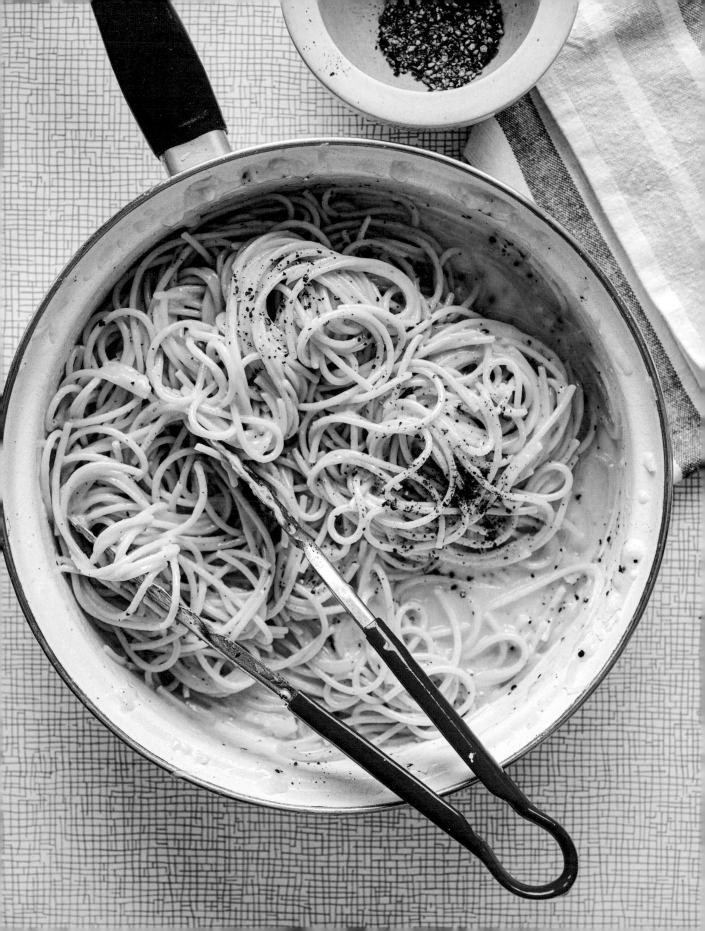

CAN'T-BE-ARSED FALAFEL

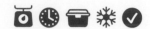

SERVES: 4
PREP: 10 minutes
COOK: 10 minutes
CALORIES: 195
DIET: VEG/V/GF/DF

Falafel, like houmous and brushing his teeth more than once a year, is one of those things that I had to spend an immeasurable amount of time persuading Paul to try. He would grimace and bluster that he didn't like the taste, texture or smell, but still I persisted because I knew one day he would crack. He always does.

To his credit, he does try. I had the luxury of coming through childhood with parents who would encourage me to try new foods at all times and then threaten to lock me under the stairs if I didn't clear my plate. As a result, I'm a cultured gastronome locked in a perennial battle with his waistline. Paul was raised entirely on Happy Shopper ready meals and nicotine (he remains the only baby to have ever come out of the womb with a roll-up behind his ear – doubly incredible when you consider how difficult it is to handle a Rizla with webbed fingers) and as a result, views anything that doesn't come with an inexplicable film of orange oil sat on top with deep suspicion.

But as I say, he does try. And, readers, so must you: this falafel is quick to make and perfect served with the raita on page 76. It doesn't look fancy in the pan, but then which of us does?

2 × 400g (14oz) tins of chickpeas, drained
100ml (3½fl oz) light coconut milk
2 cloves of garlic
25g (1oz) fresh parsley
15g (½oz) fresh coriander leaves
3 tsp ground coriander
1 tbsp ground cumin
1 tsp garam masala
zest of 1 lemon
4 tbsp lemon juice
½ tsp salt
½ tsp black pepper

Dead easy – chuck everything into a food processor and blend until smooth.

Spray the frying pan generously with oil (don't be shy) and place over a medium heat.

Add the falafel mix to the pan and gently stir until the liquid has gone and it's starting to crisp up.

Serve.

NOTES

If, like me, you like it dry and crispy, cook it for a bit longer.

Serve with rice and a nice salad.

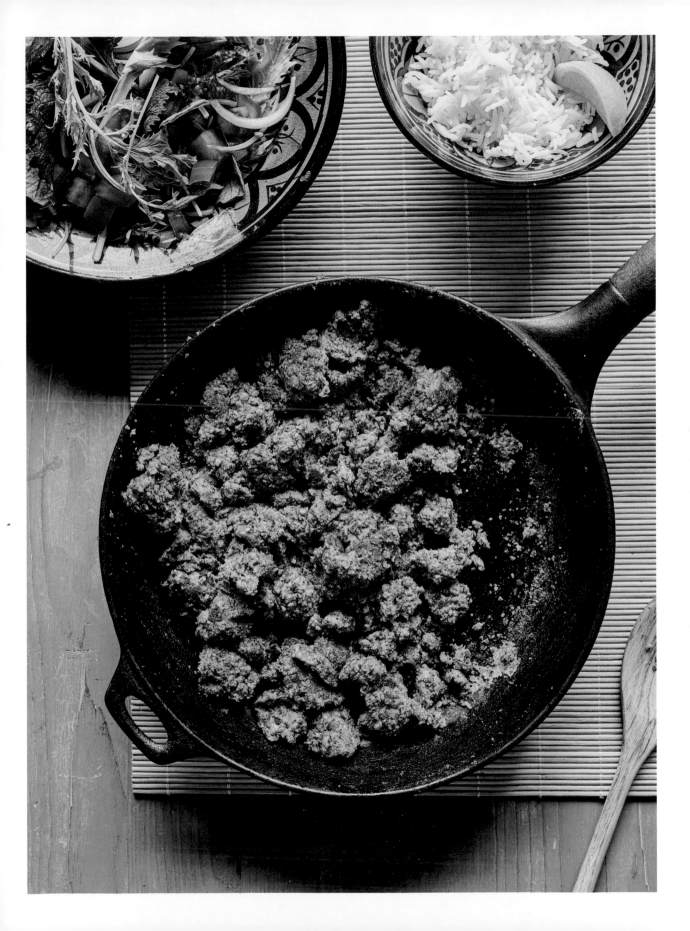

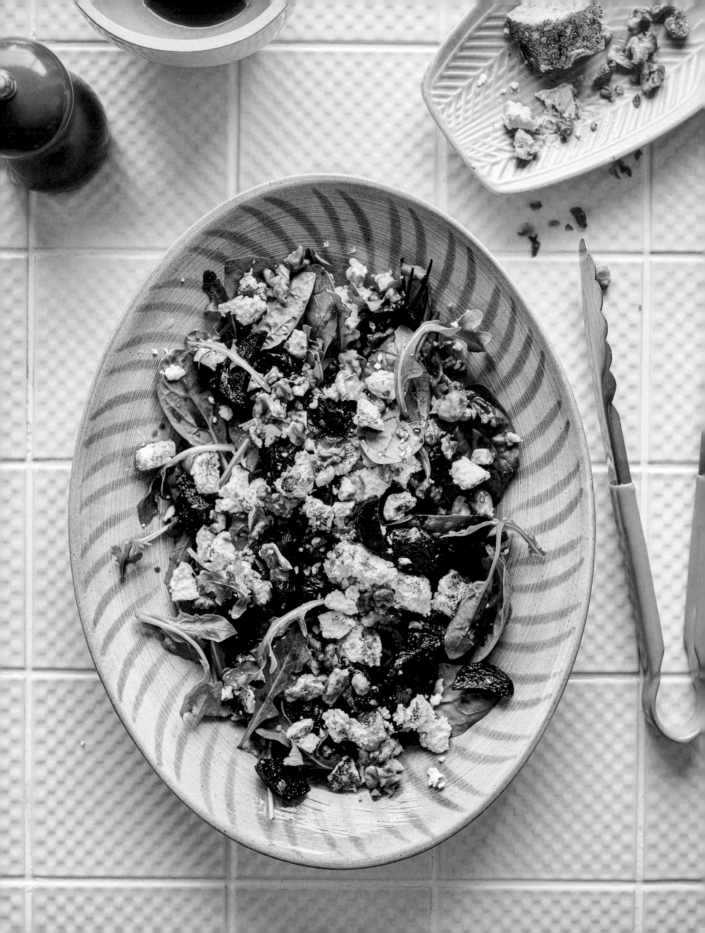

ROASTED BEETROOT SALAD

SERVES: 4
PREP: 5 minutes
COOK: 20 minutes
CALORIES: 211
DIET: VEG/GF

You know when professional idiots describe food as 'the taste of summer'? Well, they can bore off, because frankly the only thing summer tastes like to me is abject disappointment. All those people laughing gaily as they turn a lovely bronze while sipping their fancy cocktails make my blood boil, which when you consider my blood sugar levels means I'm cutting about town with strawberry jam in my veins.

I have tried to embrace the summer living ethos – this year we bought a giant hammock for the back garden. I had plans to read a book, listen to music and slowly crisp under the sun. I'd emerge from the hammock like a butterfly from a gloriously patterned chrysalis and people would gasp at the tanned Adonis before them.

Nope. The sun burned my skin as soon as I got my boobs out, and, to add insult to injury, immediately bleached my eyebrows and patches of my beard an exciting nuclear white. I looked like I'd been peering into a gas oven when it exploded. I took the hint, pushed the hammock back into the shed and went to sulkily aestivate for the next few months.

Sorry, where was I? Ah yes! This salad. Taste of summer, this.

200g (7oz) cooked beetroot
3 tbsp balsamic vinegar
1 tbsp honey
2 tsp Dijon mustard
½ tsp salt
a pinch of black pepper
400g (14oz) baby spinach
50g (1¾oz) rocket leaves
100g (3½oz) soft goat's cheese, crumbled
30g (1oz) walnuts, chopped

Preheat the oven to 200°C fan/425°F/gas mark 7.

Cut the beetroot into 1cm (½ inch) – thick slices, then cut into quarters.

Spray a baking sheet with a little oil and spread the beetroot slices on it.

Roast in the oven for 20 minutes, then remove and set aside.

Meanwhile, whisk together the balsamic vinegar, honey, mustard, salt and black pepper and set aside.

Mix together the spinach and rocket and divide between four plates.

Sprinkle over the beetroot slices, followed by the goat's cheese and walnuts.

NOTE

Pickled beetroot is perfect for this! Shake off any excess vinegar and dab dry with some kitchen paper.

SMART SWAP

Not a fan of goat's cheese? Ricotta will do.

VEGGIE MEZE

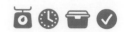

SERVES: 4
PREP: 20 minutes
COOK: 10 minutes
CALORIES: 301
DIET: VEG (check cheese is vegetarian friendly)

We can't begin to tell you the delight a meze brings us – it's like all the joy of a buffet without wondering if someone has sneezed in your taramasalata. I'd say that wasn't a euphemism, but I've met some of you. We once took part in a meze in Cyprus that saw 28 different dishes to the table. Now, we're fat of course, but goodness me even we have limits: we demurred on the last two dishes because we didn't want to look greedy. Half-inched someone's bowl of muhallebi on the way out, mind you.

If you want a more substantial dish, you could pair this up with the falafel (page 202) and the Mediterrean halloumi traybake on page 184. And, listen, we won't tell a soul if you were to slip a few sausages under the grill for snacking.

2 carrots, peeled and quartered lengthways, then halved
1 courgette, sliced
8 asparagus spears
20 cherry tomatoes
6 mini peppers
2 flatbreads, cut into wedges

For the marinade
juice of 1 lemon
2 tsp olive oil
2 tsp honey
1 tsp dried thyme
1 tsp dried rosemary
1 tsp dried parsley
1 tsp dried basil
a pinch of salt and black pepper

For the dip
150g (5½oz) reduced-fat feta cheese
80g (2¾oz) light soft cheese
1 tsp honey

In a bowl, mix together all the ingredients for the marinade.

Place all the vegetables in an ovenproof dish, pour over the marinade, and mix well.

Put the feta, soft cheese and honey into a food processor and pulse until whipped.

Preheat the grill to high.

Place the dish of veg under the grill and cook for 5–6 minutes, then turn the veg over and cook for another 5–6 minutes. Remove from the heat and set aside.

Toast the flatbreads and arrange on a plate.

Serve the vegetables with the flatbreads and the whipped feta.

> **SMART SWAP**
>
> Use whatever veg you like in this!

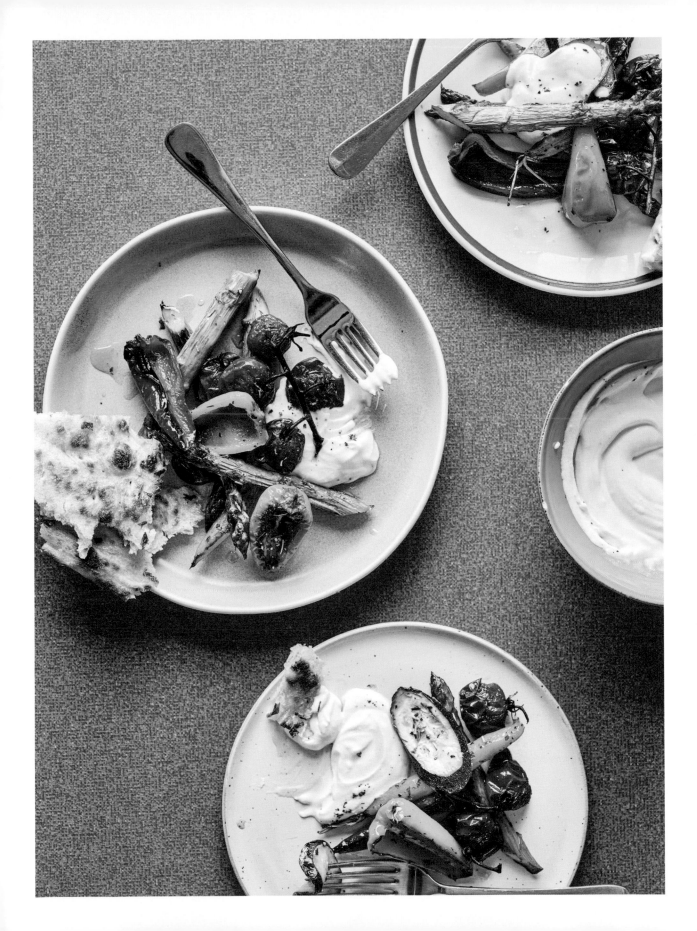

SZECHUAN MAPO DOUFU

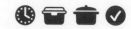

SERVES: 4
PREP: 5 minutes
COOK: 20 minutes
CALORIES: 280
DIET: VEG/V/DF

When Paul told me about this recipe – apart from me making my usual '*and a consonant please, Carol*' joke about the name – I shuddered a little at the mention of tofu, having tried several times to make it work and getting nothing but flavourless mush. I wasn't a fan.

However, he cooked it and presented it to me with that wan little face of his that screams 'love me' and won me round – not only does it work but it tastes bloody good too. I implore you not to swap it for pork unless you absolutely have to, but do use extra-firm tofu – the soft variety just won't do.

Top tip, from a tip-top bottom: get to know your local Chinese supermarkets. They have all the amazing bits you need and are so much cheaper than buying in your mainstream supermarket. There's a lovely one in Newcastle called HiYou, which I'd cheerfully recommend if you're in the area. Full disclosure: I'm partially recommending them purely because they do tasty steamed pork buns for a quid, and I've grown ever so fat on their kindness.

1 tbsp sesame oil
3 cloves of garlic, crushed
2.5cm (1 inch) ginger, finely grated
2 tbsp chilli bean paste
500g (1lb 2oz) extra-firm tofu, cubed
1 tbsp light or dark soy sauce
1 tsp hot chilli powder
1 tsp cracked black pepper
1 tsp cornflour
3 spring onions, sliced

Heat a large frying pan (or wok) over a medium-high heat and spray it with a little oil. Add the sesame oil, garlic and ginger and cook for 30 seconds, stirring constantly.

Add the chilli bean paste to the pan and cook for another minute, then add the tofu and toss to mix.

Add the soy sauce and chilli powder, along with 100ml (3½fl oz) of water. Add the black pepper and bring to the boil, then reduce the heat and simmer for 5 minutes.

Mix the cornflour with 2 tablespoons of cold water and add to the pan, then cook until the sauce starts to thicken.

Sprinkle over the sliced spring onions and serve.

NOTES

You'll find chilli bean paste in the 'World Foods' section of supermarkets – it's also called toban djan.

Serve with rice or noodles.

SMART SWAP

You can replace the tofu with diced pork to make a meaty version – cook the pork in the wok with a little oil for about 10 minutes and set aside, then put back into the pan at the same point as the tofu.

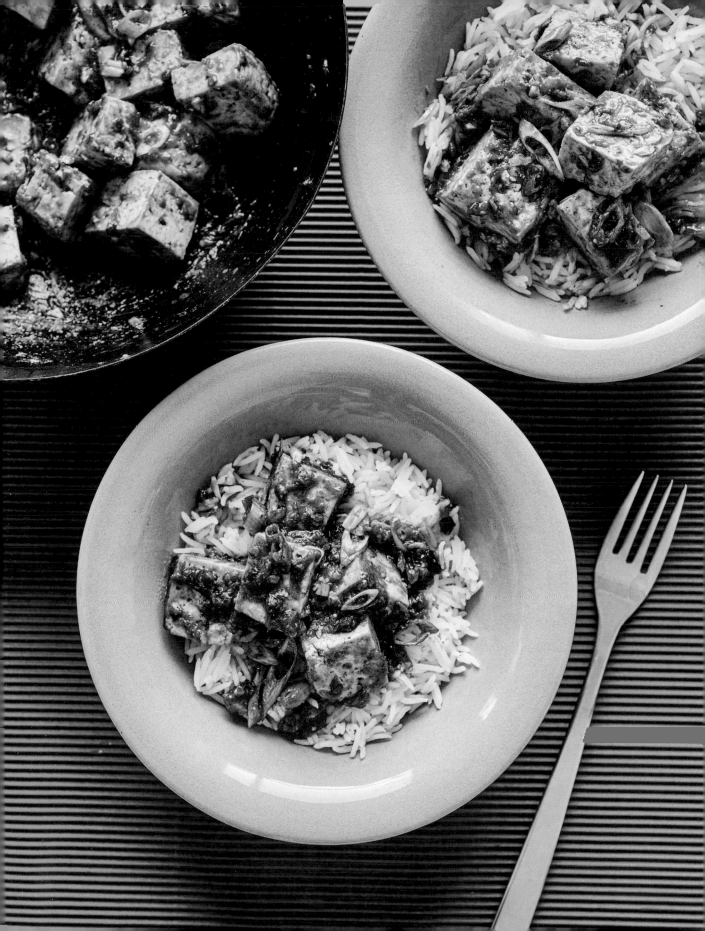

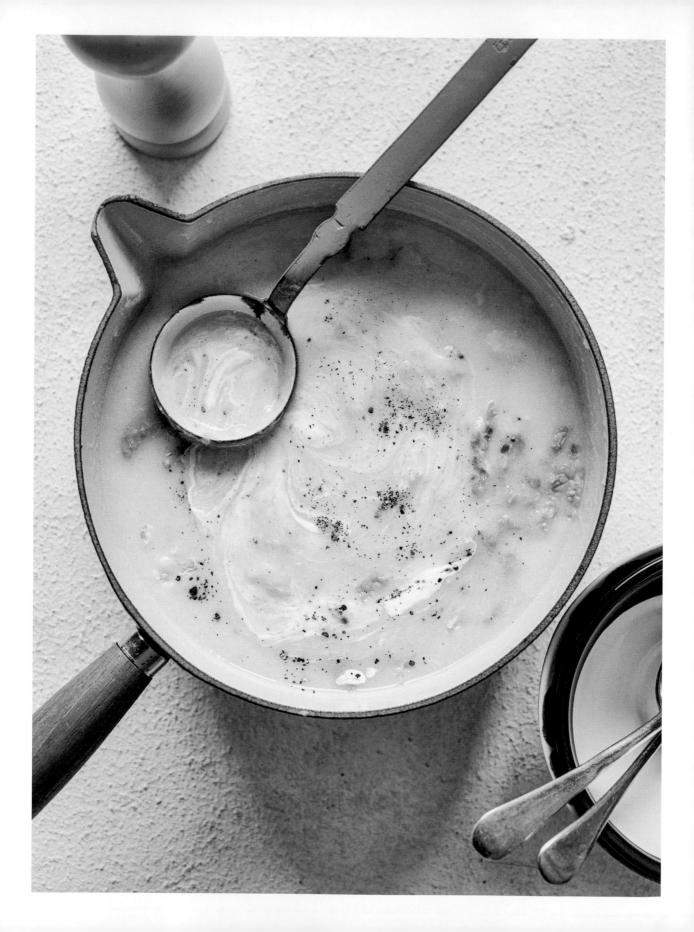

BUBBLE & SQUEAK SOUP

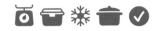

SERVES: 4
PREP: 10 minutes
COOK: 45 minutes
CALORIES: 284
DIET: VEG

30g (1oz) butter
1 onion, finely diced
½ large leek, chopped
½ Savoy cabbage, chopped
(see notes)
750g (1lb 10oz) potatoes, peeled
and chopped
1.25 litres (2¼ pints) vegetable
stock
½ tsp black pepper
350ml (12fl oz) milk
a pinch of salt

Bubble and squeak always reminds me of my dad and growing up, where every last scrap of leftovers would be used up somewhere. The evening meal after Sunday lunch would always be whatever vegetables were left, smooshed (yep) into a patty and fried, served with about eight gallons of brown sauce. It was never HP sauce, mind, we were poor: it would have been whatever knock-off variation Netto had in stock. Scandinavian for 'value', don't you know?

Sidenote: I once spent breakfast petulantly mewling that I didn't want to take my PE knickers into school in a Netto bag because people would take the piss. My mother agreed and promptly dispatched me with my sister's Tammy Girl rucksack instead. Sharp as a pin, that one.

This soup can take a lot of variation, so don't be afraid to mix it up – the addition of a sharp Cheddar at the end of cooking is something we always come back to. Perhaps you ought to give it a go.

Heat a large saucepan over a medium heat, add the butter, onion and leek and cook until the vegetables have softened.

Add the cabbage and cook for a few minutes, stirring occasionally, until the cabbage begins to wilt.

Add the potatoes, stock and black pepper to the pan and bring to a simmer. Cook for 20 minutes.

Remove from the heat and leave to cool for 5 minutes, then use a stick blender to blend until thick with a few good chunks.

Return to the heat and stir in the milk and salt, then bring to a simmer again to warm through.

Serve.

NOTES

We like to use a Savoy cabbage in this – remove the outer leaves first until you get to the 'firmer' part. A white cabbage also works well, though.

We know you're going to avoid using the butter, but don't. Trust us.

5 VEGETABLE SIDES

Sides are always a bit of a knacker when dieting, because how often do we spend an age toiling over the main dish only to forget about our bit on the side? Hell, I've been doing it for thirteen years! Here we take five simple enough sides that can be slapped on to almost any meal.

Usual rules apply: don't be limited to the vegetables we have picked out for you – the red roasted carrots work equally as well with parsnips, for example, and the best coleslaw can hold its own no matter what you mix into it. Don't be shy.

We've been making a plea to you for many years now when it comes to vegetables: keep trying new things. A friend of mine recently tried onion again for the first time in decades and it was a revelation to him. If you've been raised on tasteless, over-boiled muck then no wonder you're prejudiced against vegetables but I implore you to revisit them. Find a vegetable in the supermarket that you have no idea how to cook and then dig out a recipe you fancy – even if it is something as simple as roasting with oil, you'll really improve your options.

Also, for all that we've given you some examples of fancy sides you can make, don't ever be afraid of serving up vegetables just as they are. Fresh vegetables are wonderful and a world away from the bags of tasteless mush you get from the supermarket. By way of example, fresh peas need nothing more than a moment or two in boiling water before they're ready. Not everything needs to be gussied up, you know.

While we're here, can we recommend growing your own vegetables, whether in a tin can on a windowsill for some chillies or getting yourself an allotment to really feed the family? Allotments aren't without risk though: while most people with an allotment are terrific and friendly, there's always the danger that you'll end up next to someone with egg on their jumper, last night's dinner in their beard and no concept of 'right, well we must be getting on'. Trust us, we know.

SERVES: 4
PREP: 10 minutes
COOK: 0 minutes
CALORIES: 184
DIET: VEG (check red wine
vinegar is vegetarian friendly)

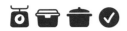 **NOTE**

Ordinary red cabbage also works
well, we just use the pickled stuff
to give it a bit of zing!

THE BEST COLESLAW

150g (5½ oz) light mayonnaise
3 tbsp red wine vinegar
1 tbsp sugar
1 tsp salt
1 tsp dried dill
½ cabbage, grated
120g pickled red cabbage, drained
   and roughly chopped
1 large carrot (4½ oz), peeled
   and grated

Whisk together the mayonnaise, red wine vinegar, sugar, salt and dill.

In a large bowl, mix together the cabbages and the carrot and pour over
the dressing.

Toss and serve.

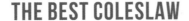

SERVES: 4
PREP: 10 minutes
COOK: 30 minutes
CALORIES: 240
DIET: VEG/V/GF/DF

HASSELBACK POTATOES

8 medium potatoes
2 tbsp olive oil
4 cloves of garlic, crushed
1 tbsp finely chopped fresh parsley
salt and pepper

Preheat the oven to 200°C/425°F/gas mark 7.

Place the handles of two wooden spoons either side of a potato – the
trick here is that it'll act as a guide to stop you slicing all the way through.

Gently take a sharp knife and cut thin slices through the potatoes –
make sure not to slice all the way.

Mix together the olive oil and garlic and use a pastry brush to brush
over the potatoes.

Place the potatoes onto a baking tray and bake in the oven for
30 minutes, basting occasionally with any oil that runs off into the tray.

Remove from the oven and sprinkle over the parsley, salt and pepper.

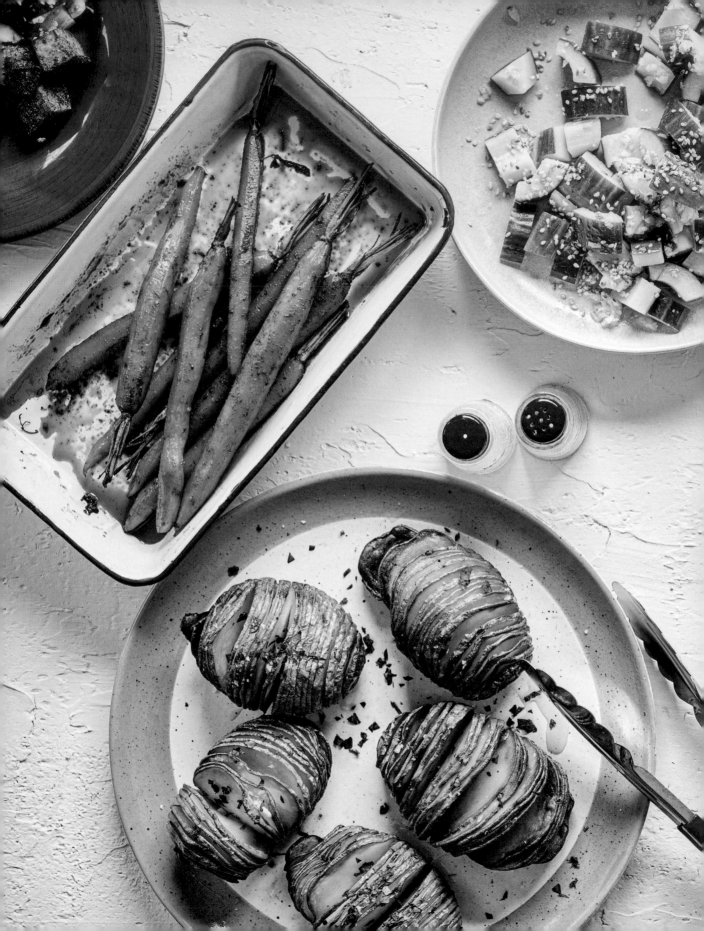

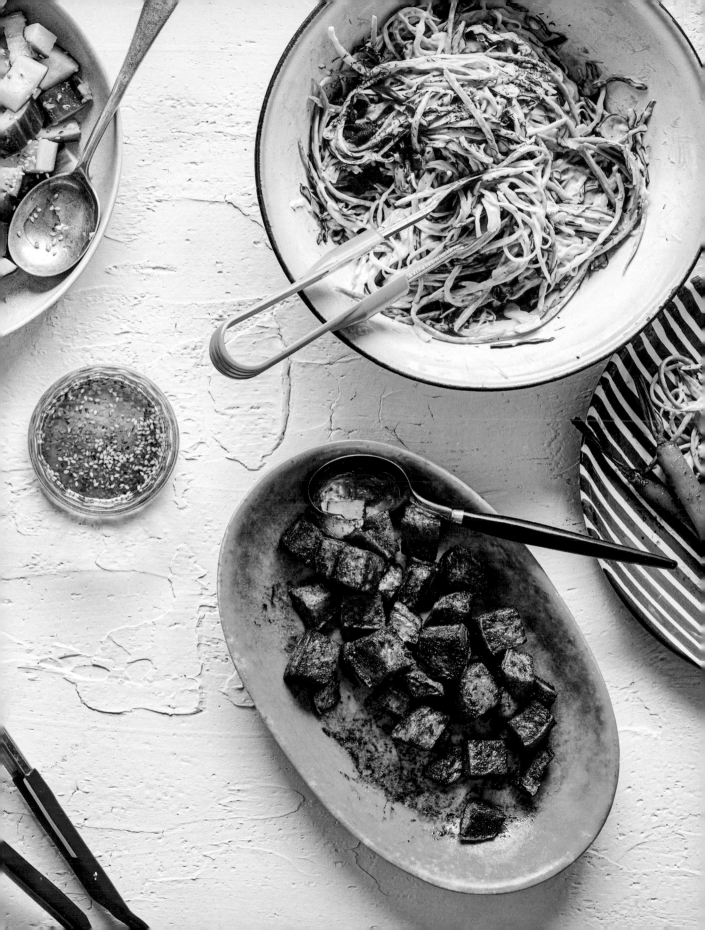

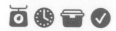

SERVES: 4
PREP: 25 minutes
COOK: 0 minutes
CALORIES: 69
DIET: VEG/V/GF/DF

NOTE

This is great as a side on its own or as part of a big salad to help sexy up the usually boring cucumber.

CUCUMBER SALAD

1 cucumber
1 tsp salt
1 tsp sugar

For the dressing
½ tsp salt
½ tsp sugar
1½ tbsp rice vinegar
1 tbsp sesame oil
2 garlic cloves, crushed
1cm (½ inch) ginger, grated
2 tsp sesame seeds

Slice the cucumber in half lengthways, scrape out the seeds using a teaspoon and chuck away.

Dice the cucumber into 2cm (¾ inch) pieces.

Sprinkle with the salt and sugar and set aside for 20 minutes.

Meanwhile, whisk together all of the dressing ingredients.

Gently toss the cucumber with the dressing and serve.

SERVES: 4
PREP: 5 minutes
COOK: 40 minutes
CALORIES: 88
DIET: VEG/GF/DF

NOTE

The long, skinny carrots are best for this.

RED ROASTED CARROTS

1 tbsp honey
1 tsp hot chilli powder
1 tbsp olive oil
1 tsp salt
½ tsp paprika
1 bunch of carrots

Preheat the oven to 190°C/410°F/gas mark 7.

In a bowl, mix together the honey, chilli powder, olive oil, salt and paprika.

Pour over the carrots and toss well to coat.

Roast in the oven for 20 minutes, turn, then roast for another 20 minutes.

Serve.

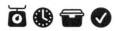

ROASTED SWEET POTATOES

SERVES: 4
PREP: 5 minutes
COOK: 25 minutes
CALORIES: 168
DIET: VEG/V/GF/DF

NOTE

Well, all right, peel if you want but they're so much better with!

2 large sweet potatoes
1 tbsp olive oil
2 cloves of garlic, crushed
1 tsp paprika
1 tsp cumin

Preheat the oven to 220°C/475°F/gas mark 8.

Wash the potatoes and dice into 2.5cm (1 inch) cubes (don't peel!).

Gently toss in the olive oil, garlic, paprika and cumin.

Spread out onto a baking sheet and bake for 15 minutes.

Gently turn, then bake for another 10 minutes.

Serve.

EASY SUN-DRIED TOMATO PASTA

SERVES: 4
PREP: 5 minutes
COOK: 15 minutes
CALORIES: 229
DIET: VEG/V/DF

It does seem that we come back to sun-dried tomato pasta ever so much, but it's Paul's go-to lunch and he spends so long perfecting the bugger that we must pay him lip service and include it. Which is curious, because I only tend to pay him lip service on his birthday or when I've been indiscreet.

When we say use any pasta you like, we mean it – it really doesn't matter in a dish like this. Whatever you have in, use! I say that with a pause: can you recall there was a shortage on pasta and loo rolls not so long since, when idiots rushed out and bought a metric tonne of tagliatelle because they thought the end of the world was nigh? Well, as a result, we struggled to find pasta and had to make do with a packet of penis pasta that had been gifted to us by a friend. Best part? No bugger noticed that our pan of sloppy joe reshoot was awash with tiny little willies.

But you know what? It still tasted good! So if you're feeling especially fruity, feel free to make this with some explicit pasta and send us the results via social media. We promise to laugh politely at at least three of them.

200g (7oz) pasta of your choice
½ onion, finely diced
3 cloves of garlic, crushed
8 sun-dried tomatoes, chopped
1 tomato, finely chopped
1 tbsp dried mixed herbs
1 tsp dried chilli flakes

Cook the pasta according to the packet instructions, then drain.

Spray a large pan with a little oil and place it over a medium heat.

Add the onion and cook for 1 minute, then add the garlic and cook for another 30 seconds.

Add all the other ingredients and cook for another 5 minutes.

Toss with the pasta and serve.

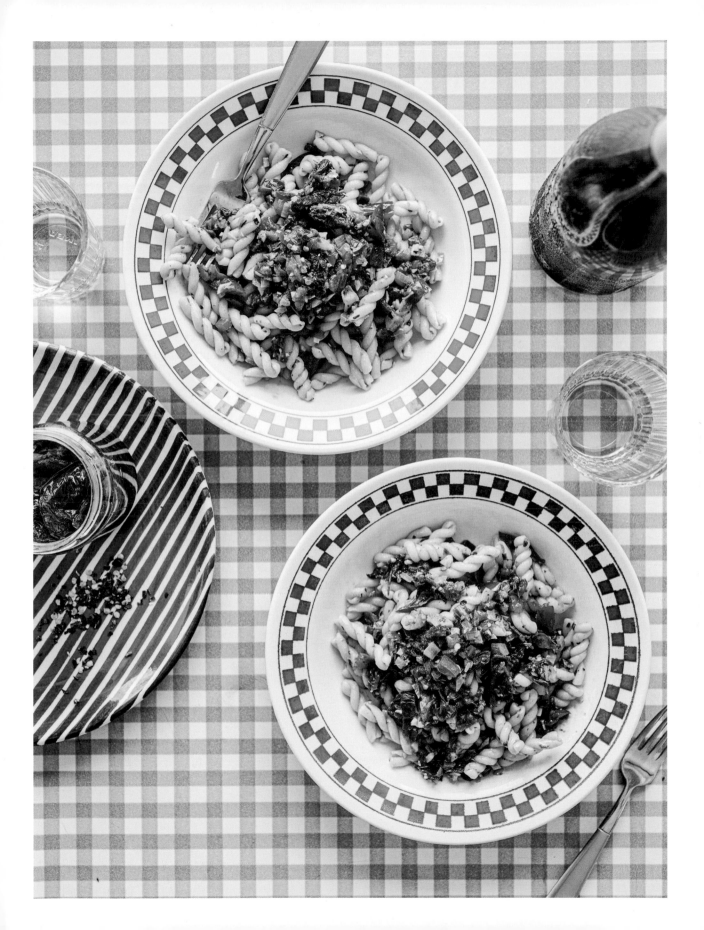

SUPER-SIMPLE BRUSCHETTA

SERVES: 4
PREP: 10 minutes
COOK: 8 minutes
CALORIES: 357
DIET: VEG/V/DF
(check balsamic is vegan friendly)

There's a lot to be said for simple food, and hence this bruschetta is making an appearance here. Remember, there's a world of flavoured oils out there, so if you're looking to jazz this up a bit, take your pick. Also, a further tip: cover this in cheese and you've got proper fancy cheese on toast.

The first time we made this was in a windswept caravan in some desolate wasteland off the North Sea. It was a rough weekend, I can't lie: an exercise in trying to shake money from my pockets at every given opportunity. Across the way were a family whose neighbours would probably describe them as 'rough diamonds' but only so they didn't get their windows put through and their bins shat in, and boy were they loud.

Not the fun loud, mind: no raucous laughter or good-time noise, just endless shouting. I've never seen a Pot Noodle cooked via the medium of yelling before. As a result, they kept us awake until half three. Luckily, we woke them via the medium of seagulls at 4.30 a.m. because it turns out that taking the leftover baguette from this recipe and hurling it on top of the neighbour's caravan attracts all the seagulls within a ten-mile radius to clatter and tatter all over their roof.

Honestly, the words we heard – you'd blush. To the food!

1 small baguette, sliced
5 tomatoes, chopped
2 cloves of garlic, crushed
20 fresh basil leaves, finely chopped
1 tsp salt
1 tsp dried oregano
2 tbsp balsamic vinegar

Preheat the oven to 180°C fan/400°F/gas mark 6.

Lay the bread on a baking sheet and spray it with a little oil.

Bake in the oven for 6–8 minutes, until slightly golden, then remove and leave to cool.

Meanwhile, mix gently together the tomatoes, garlic, basil leaves, salt and oregano.

Spoon the tomato mixture on to the bread and drizzle over the balsamic vinegar.

NOTE

This is perfect as a starter, side or even as a lunch! Add some diced onion if you want to make it go even further.

SMART SWAP

We use a baguette as it gives the best crunch, but ordinary toast will do the trick just as well.

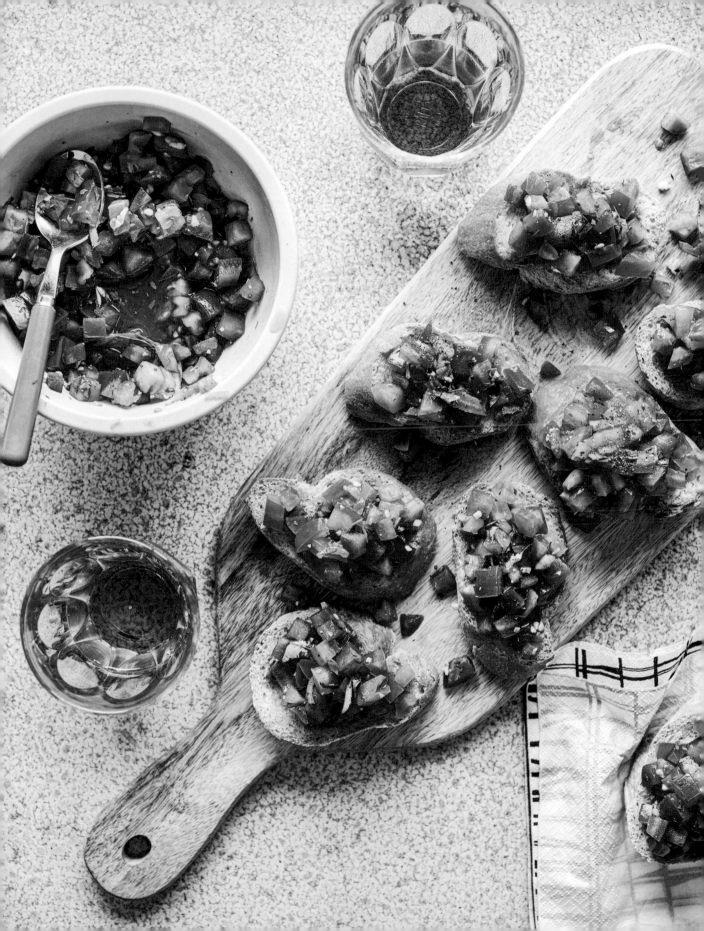

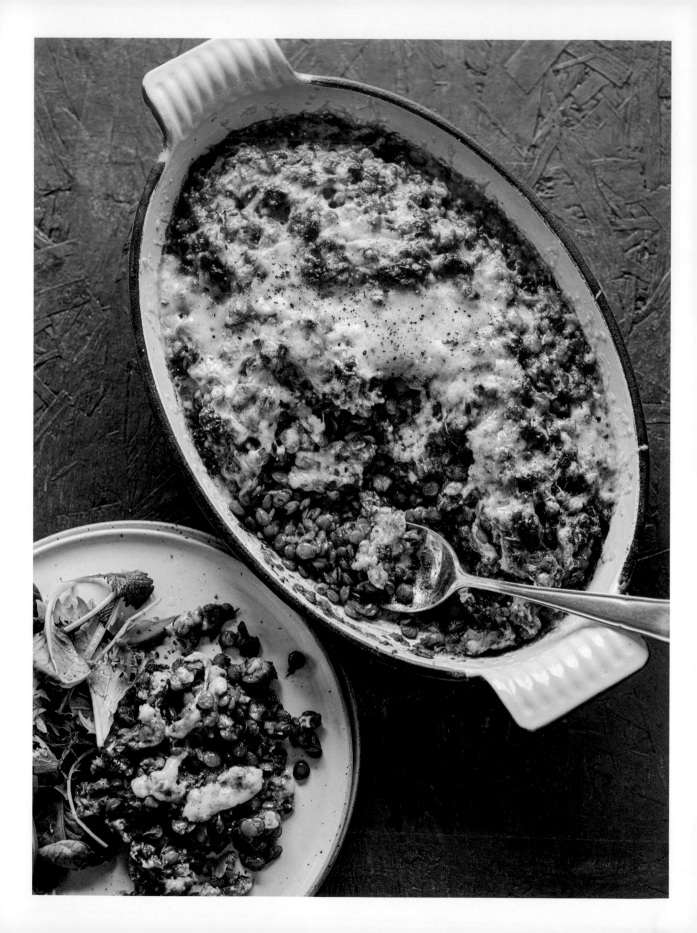

CHEESY LENTIL BAKE

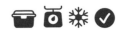

SERVES: 4
PREP: 5 minutes
COOK: 45 minutes
CALORIES: 499
DIET: VEG (check cheese is vegetarian friendly)

A lentil bake always makes me think of Mary, my old flatmate, who made them often.

Mary was wonderful but exhausting: she would change her persuasions as often as I changed my bedsheets (which back in the day of youthful exuberance was surprisingly often). I'd come home for her to announce she was vegan and thus had dragged our crappy leather sofa into the back lane, as it was 'cruel'. Two days later, she'd be snaffling through a box of chicken without a moment of guilt.

In between the screaming, throwing things at the wall, shrieking and crying – with occasional input from Mary, too – we had so much fun. Alas, she moved away when I shacked up with Paul and we drifted apart. If you're out there, flower, get in touch.

400g (14oz) dried green or brown lentils
6 cloves of garlic, finely chopped
2 tsp paprika
1 tsp cayenne pepper
1 tsp garam masala
4 tbsp tomato purée
2 tsp dried tarragon
2 tsp dried rosemary
250g (9oz) low-fat cheese, grated
20g (¾oz) vegetarian Italian hard cheese, grated

Rinse the lentils in a sieve under cold water, then place in a pan with plenty of fresh water. Bring to a simmer and cook for 20 minutes, until tender, then drain and set aside.

Preheat the oven to 220°C fan/475°F/gas mark 9.

Spray a large ovenproof frying pan or casserole dish with a little oil and place over a medium heat. Add the garlic and fry for a minute or two. Add the paprika, cayenne pepper and garam masala and stir well.

Reduce the heat to medium-low, add the tomato purée and stir again.

Add the lentils to the pan along with 100ml (3½fl oz) of water and stir well. When it begins to simmer, add the tarragon and rosemary and remove from the heat.

Spread the grated cheeses on top and bake in the oven for 15 minutes.

NOTES

We love this with roast potatoes, but honestly, have whatever you like with it!

This tastes even better warmed up the next day – take some to work for lunch!

EASY LEMON RICE

SERVES: 4
PREP: 5 minutes
COOK: 10 minutes
CALORIES: 224
DIET: VEG/V/DF

We call this lemon rice, despite it also having lime in it – as lies go, it's akin to calling obviously grilled meat steamed hams. That's a reference that'll probably land for about 10% of our readers, and that's good enough for us.

We had this rice on a flight back from Tokyo – we had managed to acquire so many air miles by furnishing our house entirely using a credit card that we were able to travel there and back in first class. It was tremendous, even if we did feel like fish out of water. Neither of us are fancy folk, but damn if I didn't feel superb sitting there in seat 1A with my XL pyjamas spread over my 3XL frame.

About halfway into the flight, I decided this was the time for Paul and I to join the mile-high club. I'm already a member thanks to a frisky and persistent ex, but Paul is very much by the book and doesn't like to break rules. Nevertheless, buoyed up by far too much gin and champagne, I slipped him a note to 'meet me in the loo for some action'.

His response back? 'It would be like moving two settees in a lift, so I think the fuck not.'

Poor sport.

200g (7oz) basmati rice
¾ tsp mustard powder
2 tbsp chopped dry-roasted
    peanuts
½ tsp ground turmeric
zest of 1 lime
2 green chillies, finely diced
2 lemons

Rinse the rice and cook according to the packet instructions, then drain and set aside.

Spray a large frying pan with a little oil and place over a high heat. Add the mustard powder and peanuts and stir.

Add the turmeric, lime zest and green chillies and stir well, then cook for 1 minute.

Remove the pan from the heat and stir in the cooked rice.

Squeeze in the juice from the lemons and stir well.

NOTE

If you're in a rush, the microwave pouches of rice are perfect for this – use two of them.

SMART SWAP

You can replace the peanuts with cashews if you prefer, or leave them out.

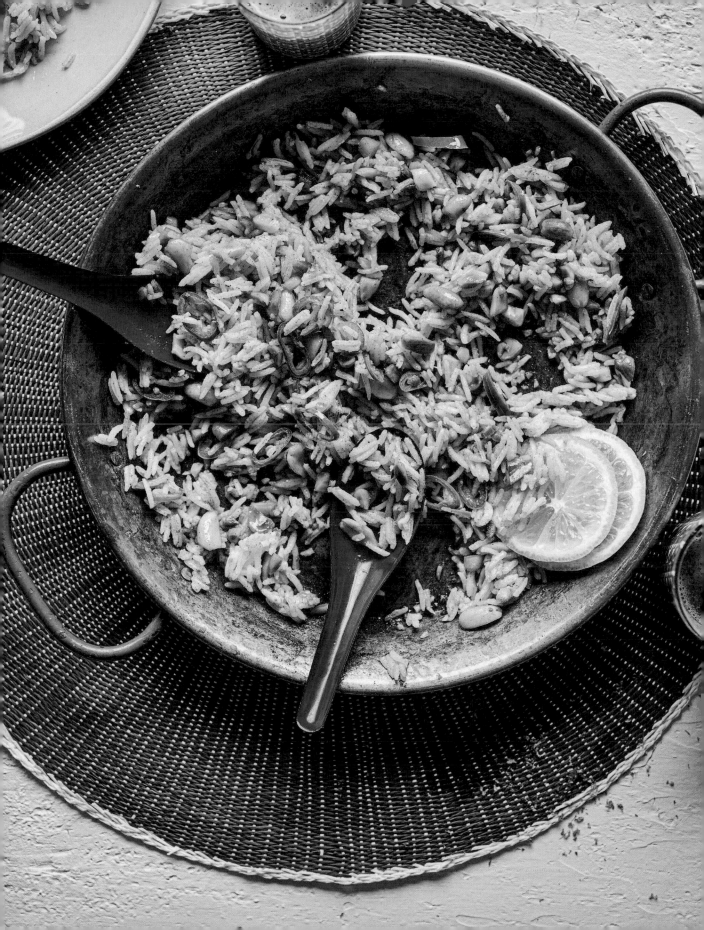

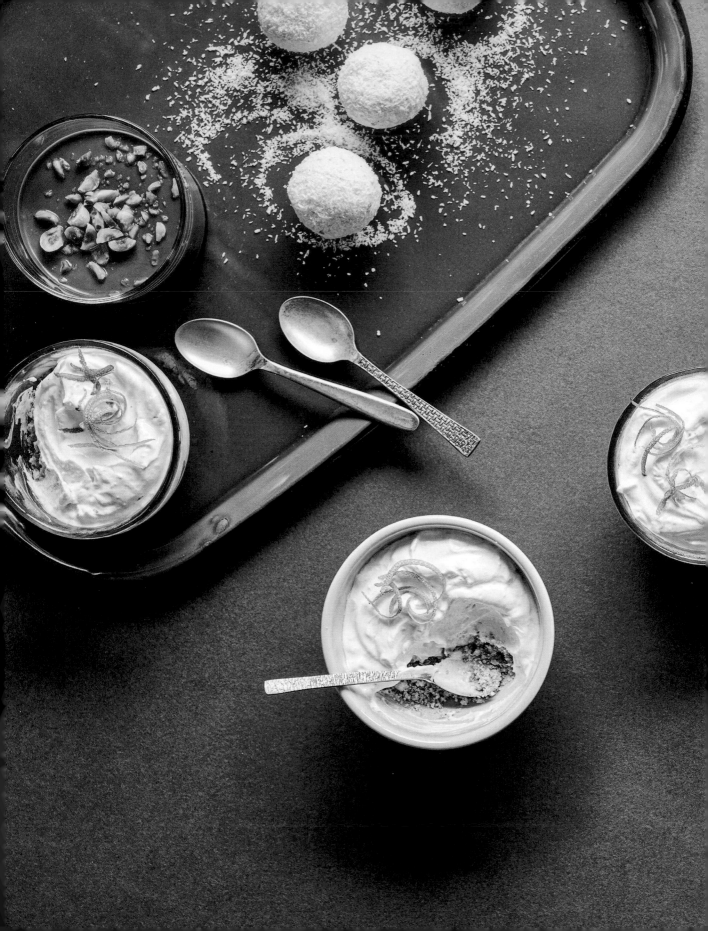

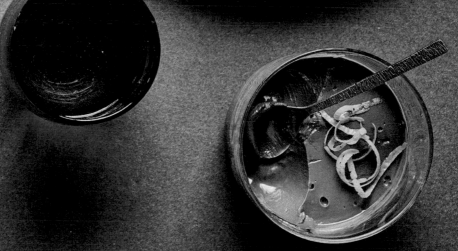

SWEETS
& TREATS

CRACKLE-TOP STRAWBERRY JELLY POTS

SERVES: 4
PREP: 20 minutes
(plus about 7 hours setting)
COOK: 0 minutes
CALORIES: 228
DIET: GF

Looking for a low-calorie yet fancy dessert? This is the one. It comes with a tale about living with health anxiety, something I touched on in our last book. I won't talk more about it here, only to say I'm still doing fine. That's many years in a row now, and I used to think the darkness would never lift. If you're reading this in the same position, I hope it provides you with some comfort to know it absolutely gets better.

But, if we're not going to take a moment to look at our shoes and tug our forelocks, what is this for? A simple message, really – just try to be a decent person. I'm a raving cynic when it comes to life, but for the last few months I have tried to be more understanding and patient and it has calmed me down. Some people wear their bitchiness on their sleeves as a badge of honour and it is a poisonous trait indeed.

So, try to be the opposite. We shouldn't need to be corralled into being kind by a hashtag campaign, but it sure felt better when that happened. Indeed, be like this dessert: sweet on the outside, creamy in the middle and fruity in the bottom. Always served me well.

1 sachet of no-added-sugar jelly
12 tbsp fat-free vanilla yoghurt
100g (3½oz) strawberries
80g (2¾oz) milk chocolate
a few fresh mint leaves

Make up the jelly according to the packet instructions, and pour into four glasses or bowls. Put into the fridge and leave to set for about 6 hours.

Once set, top up the bowls or glasses with vanilla yoghurt and put back into the fridge.

Chop the strawberries, put them into a pan with a little hot water, and heat gently until the fruit has broken down and thickened a little. Put them into a bowl in the fridge for later.

Meanwhile, break the chocolate into a bowl and gently warm in the microwave until melted.

Remove the bowls from the fridge and gently pour the melted chocolate on top. It's best to drizzle it over the back of a hot spoon to avoid it mixing too much with the yoghurt – you want it to sit on top.

Put back into the fridge and leave to set for an hour. Top with the strawberries and a few fresh mint leaves and serve.

NOTE

If you're feeling fancy – as we frequently are – tip the glasses at a 45° angle when you add the jelly – it adds a nice diagonal effect.

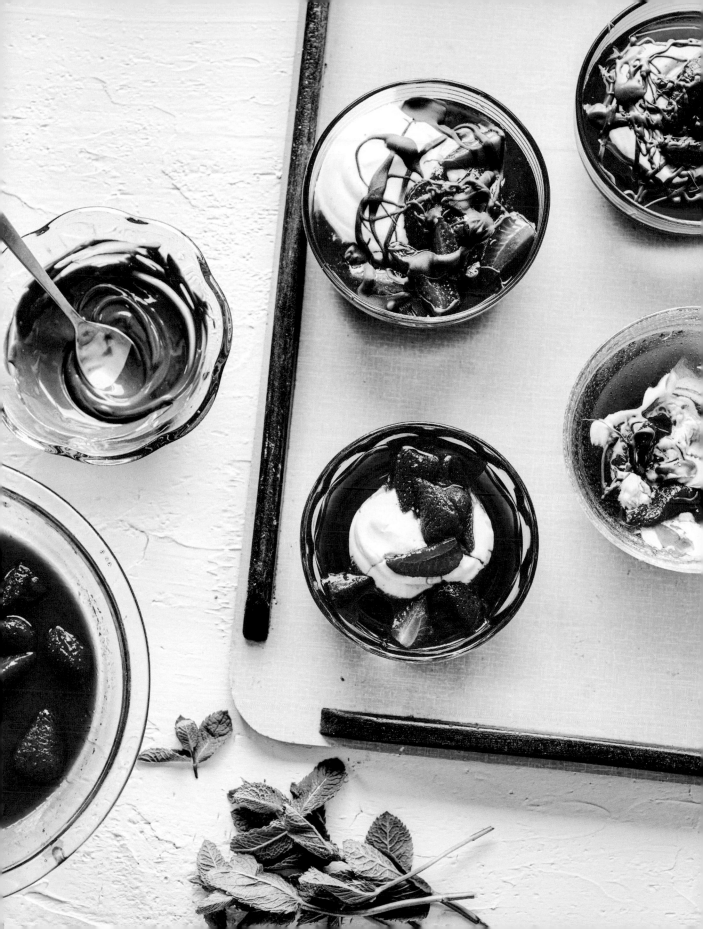

ACTUALLY PRETTY DECENT MUG CAKE

SERVES: 1
PREP: 5 minutes
COOK: 1 minute
CALORIES: 497
DIET: VEG

Look: we're putting this entry in under severe duress. Not because the recipe itself is anything other than utterly delightful – this is us, after all – but because we're firm believers that if you're going to treat yourself, you're better off having a wedge of something delicious. As we've mentioned before, cakes need flour, fat and eggs to work properly, but that doesn't stop you all trying your hardest to make a 'slimming version'.

You have no idea of the mental toll it puts on a man to witness these abominations served up in the name of dieting: cakes that look like something you'd pick off your knee three days after falling off your bike, with about as much taste profile as a bail hostel blanket. So we experimented with how to make a decent cake-in-a-mug as a compromise. The first few attempts without sugar were frankly, bloody awful. I would prefer to eat my own face than go there again.

However, we think we've cracked it. This isn't going to win many awards for presentation, but as a halfway point between eating your feelings and enjoying yourself, it works. Don't be tempted to skip any ingredient – the sum of this cake is very much in the sum of its parts.

Enjoy!

¼ tsp instant coffee granules
2 tbsp milk
2 tbsp plain flour
2 tbsp brown sugar
4 tsp cocoa powder
¼ tsp baking powder
a pinch of salt
3 tsp vegetable oil
½ tsp vanilla extract
10g (¼oz) dark chocolate chips

Mix the coffee granules with the milk until dissolved.

In a mug, using a fork, mix together the flour, sugar, cocoa powder, baking powder and salt.

Pour the coffee mix into the mug along with the oil and vanilla, and give it a good stir.

Gently stir in the chocolate chips.

Microwave on high for 1 minute (if it's still a bit boggy, whack on for another 10 seconds).

NOTE

All right, it's not gonna be the best, but for those times where you REALLY want a cake, this will hit the spot nicely, and is ACTUALLY a proper cake rather than an omelette.

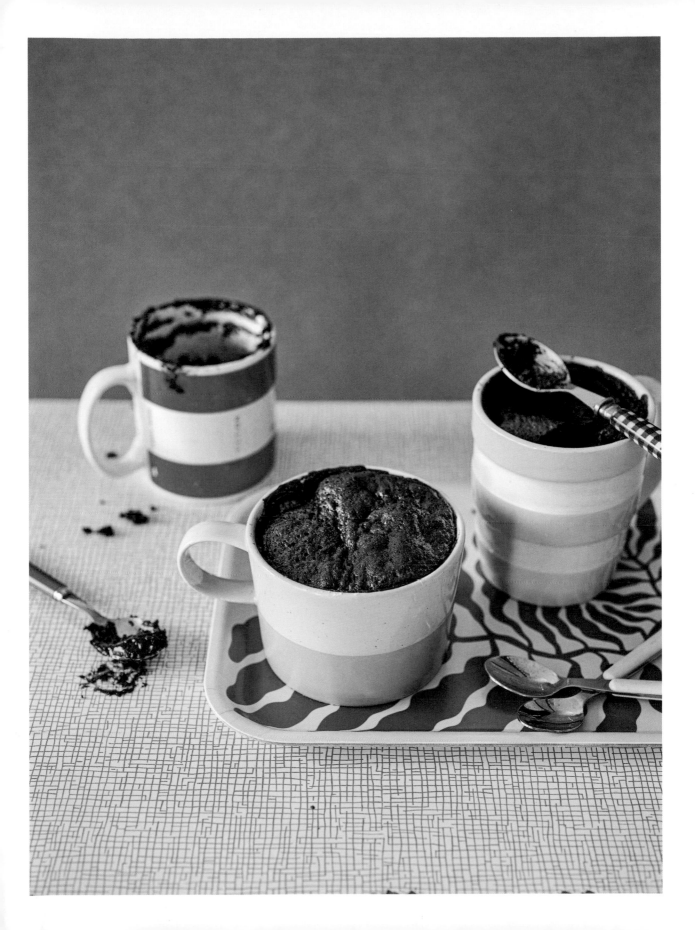

KEY LIME PIE CHEESECAKE

SERVES: 4
PREP: 30 minutes
COOK: 10 minutes (plus about 20 minutes setting)
CALORIES: 294
DIET: VEG

8 digestive biscuits, roughly crumbled
300g (10½oz) Greek yoghurt
200g (7oz) light soft cheese
1 tbsp granulated sugar
1 tbsp lime zest
3 tbsp lime juice

You'll need to forgive us: this is very much a rough and ready cheesecake rather than the extravagant dish you might pick up in a fancy restaurant. I say fancy: Paul and I rarely eat out anywhere where they don't have a colouring-in section on the back of the menu. Indeed, this is something we tend to order when we go to our pub quiz on a Thursday evening. It's held in one of those pubs where unless you're local you will enter through the door and leave out the window, but we love it – it's quite a warming feeling to be the only person in the room with a full set of teeth.

Do love a pub quiz though: between the four of us, we have most specialities covered. I'm good with cinema and science, Paul has music and cooking nailed down, and between them, Patrick and Andrew have literature and history in the bag. Embarrassingly and slightly playing to stereotype, we all fall down on sports questions. What can I say? I spent all my teenage PE lessons lusting after the teacher with his tree-trunk legs because I was nothing but a terrible slattern even then.

Paul doesn't like to add butter to the biscuits when making the base, but I encourage you to do so if you can spare the calories. Also, I prefer to use ginger nuts rather than digestives, but hey: I'll let you decide.

Divide the crumbled biscuits between four glasses or bowls.

Using a hand mixer, whisk together the yoghurt and soft cheese until smooth. Add the sugar, lime zest and juice and whisk until smooth.

Spoon the mixture into the glasses or bowls and leave to set in the fridge for 20 minutes.

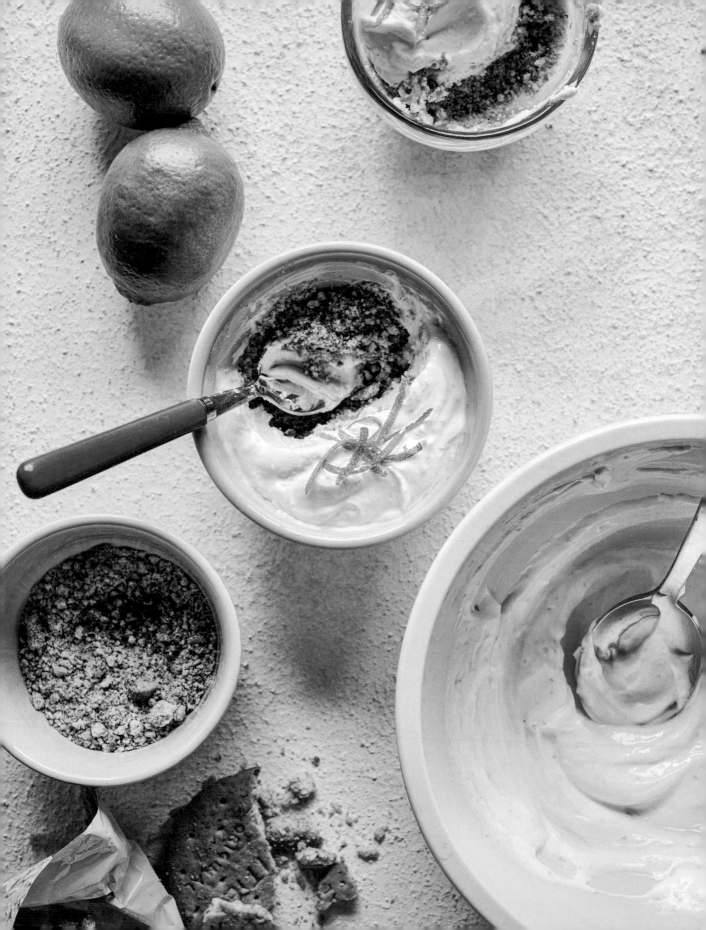

5 QUICK SLIM COCKTAILS

You'll need to forgive us these indulgences, but there's a hidden trio who keep the twochubbycubs train rolling along. We gave them a tip of our hat in the last book, but we've decided to go all in on buttering them up. Our fabulous moderators – Jeanette Armour, Vicky McDermott and Lisa-Clare Fairbairn – keep an eye on our group when we're torn away by fire and flood, and we truly couldn't do without them. We've immortalized them in three light cocktails – stuff we drink when we want to calm our shakes but not overdo the calories – and we're sure you can find something in here you'll love. We've included two more because we're a big fan of the number five here.

SERVES: 1
CALORIES: 175
DIET: VEG/V/GF/DF

THE JEANETTE

200ml (7fl oz) Irn Bru
50ml (1¾fl oz) gin
a slice of orange (to garnish)

Mix together.

Cause a scene.

SERVES: 1
CALORIES: 221
DIET: VEG/GF/DF

THE STICKY VICKY

50ml (1¾fl oz) vodka
25ml (1fl oz) St Germain
25ml (1fl oz) fresh lime juice
1 tsp honey
a handful of ice cubes
a slice of lime (to garnish)

Shake everything except the garnish in a cocktail shaker.

Serve over ice with a slice of lime.

THE LIL' LISA

SERVES: 1
CALORIES: 221
DIET: VEG/V/GF/DF
(check champagne
is vegetarian friendly)

4 raspberries
50ml (1¾fl oz) Chambord
100ml (3½fl oz) champagne
    (or prosecco)

Gently crush the raspberries and put them into a champagne flute.

Add the Chambord and top with the champagne.

CHUBBY MARGARITA

SERVES: 1
CALORIES: 140
DIET: VEG/V/GF/DF

120ml (4½fl oz) lime juice
50ml (1¾fl oz) tequila
50ml (1¾fl oz) orange juice
a handful of ice cubes

Put everything into a blender and process until slushy.

FIZZY DIZZY ORANGE

SERVES: 1
CALORIES: 268
DIET: VEG/V/GF/DF

200ml (7fl oz) fresh orange juice
50ml (1¾fl oz) vodka
25ml (1fl oz) triple sec
a handful of ice cubes
60ml (2¼fl oz) soda water
a slice of orange (to garnish)

Chuck everything except the soda water and the garnish into a cocktail shaker and give it a good go. Pour into a glass, stir in the soda water and add a slice of orange.

NOTE

For cocktail recipe images, please see overleaf on p236-237 (appearing from left to right across the double page: THE STICKY VICKY, CHUBBY MARGARITA, THE JEANETTE, THE LIL' LISA, FIZZY DIZZY ORANGE). I know, we don't miss a trick!

SWEETS & TREATS

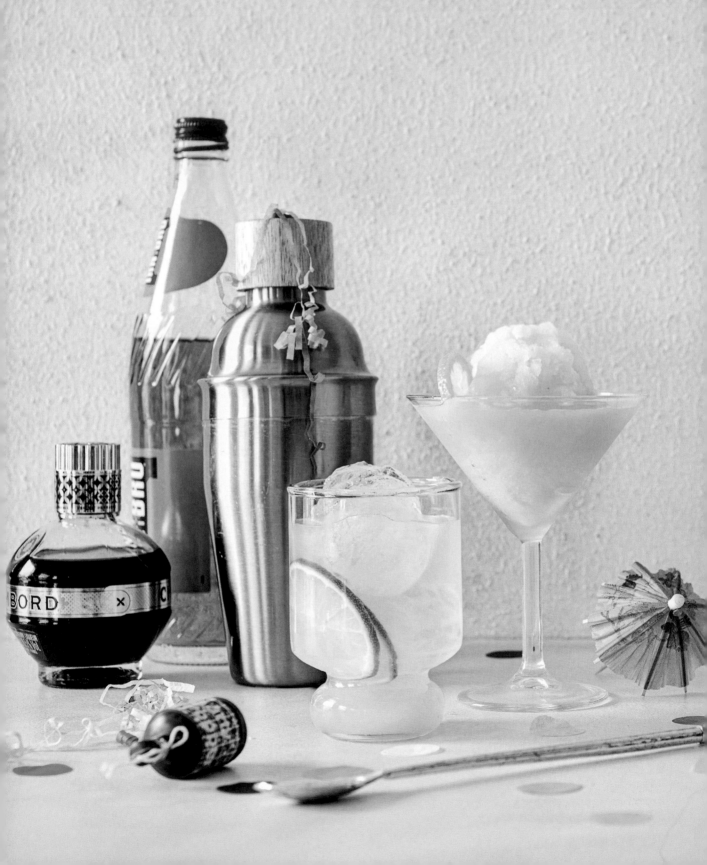

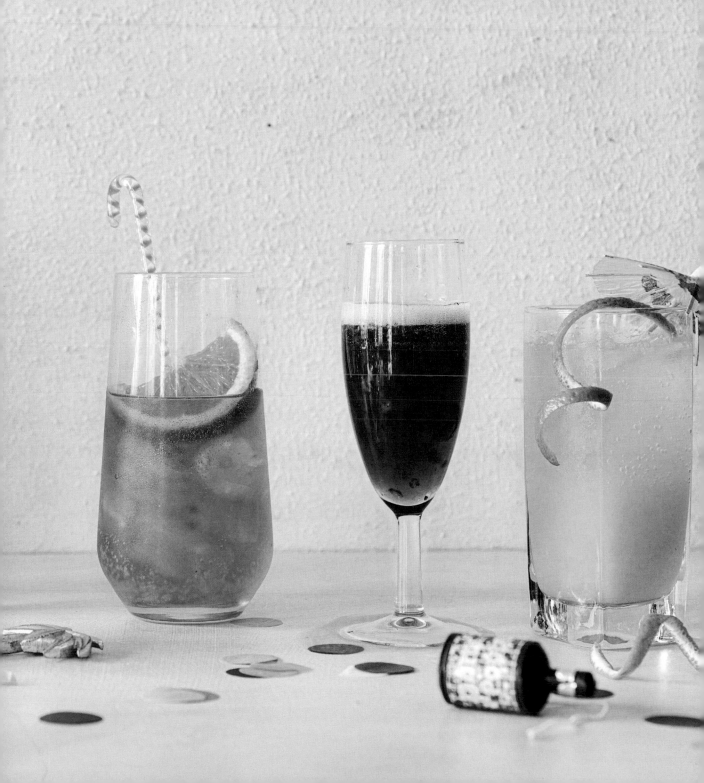

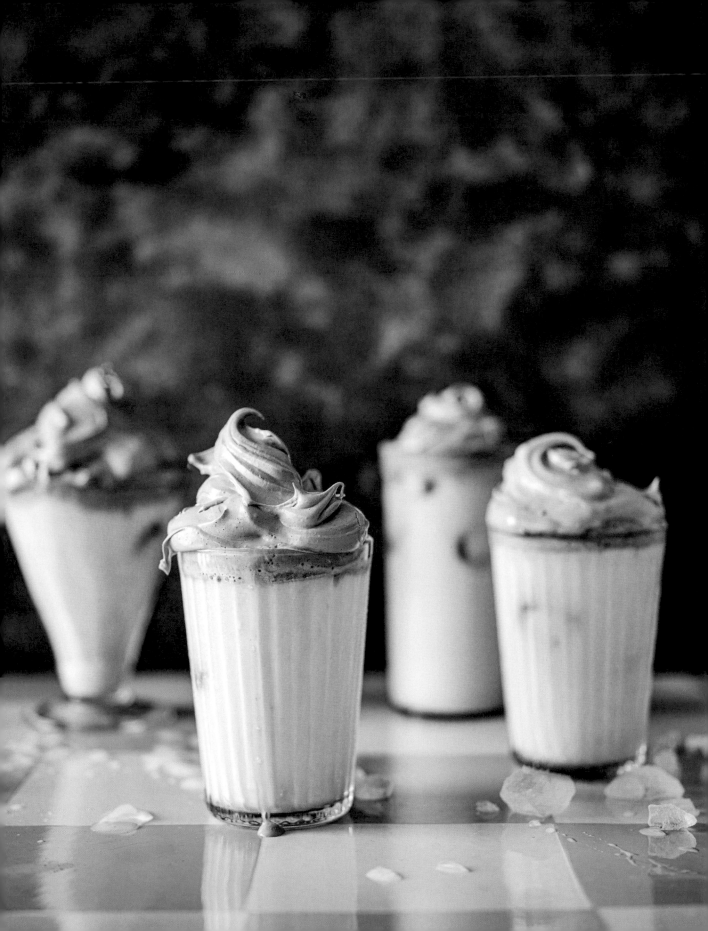

DALGONA

SERVES: 4
PREP: 10 minutes
COOK: 0 minutes
CALORIES: 100
DIET: VEG/V/DF/GF

It took every fibre of my being not to call this 'Dalgona – I barely knew 'er', repeating a joke I used in the last book where everything with an 'ah' sound is immediately suffixed by the 'barely knew her' line. It's not a great joke, but damn it, it's one of ours. I do wonder what on Earth people must think of Paul and me when they see us out and about – we're always laughing and shrieking at utter nonsense that means nothing to anyone else. But every couple has their in-jokes, surely?

For example, Paul does a mean impression, and one thing he will often shout at me is his hot-take on Janice Battersby from old *Coronation Street*. One shriek of 'LEEEEEES' at me is enough to send me into paroxysms of giggles. Similarly, we watched an episode of *Wife Swap* right at the start of the relationship and about 80 per cent of our current catchphrases come from that. I'm not saying we're outdated, but when your comedy comes from some rough bird from Barnsley shouting at her kids back in 2005 …

… Luckily, we do embrace current fads, and this is where the dalgona recipe comes from. When it started appearing on Instagram I dismissed it as a flash in the pan that would fizzle out, like planking or healthy eating. But no – it lives on – and this is our take on it. It's a genuinely tasty wee drink and if you don't try it, it clearly means you hate us.

4 tbsp granulated sugar
4 tbsp instant coffee
4 tbsp hot water
a good handful of ice cubes
280ml (9½fl oz) almond milk

In a bowl, whisk together the sugar, coffee and hot water until thick and light.

Fill four glasses with ice cubes and top with the almond milk.

Spoon over the thick coffee mixture.

NOTES

A hand or stand mixer is best for this! You're after stiff peaks.

The amount of sugar might seem shocking but it's worth it – this makes a great refreshing dessert or snack! Don't let it put you off.

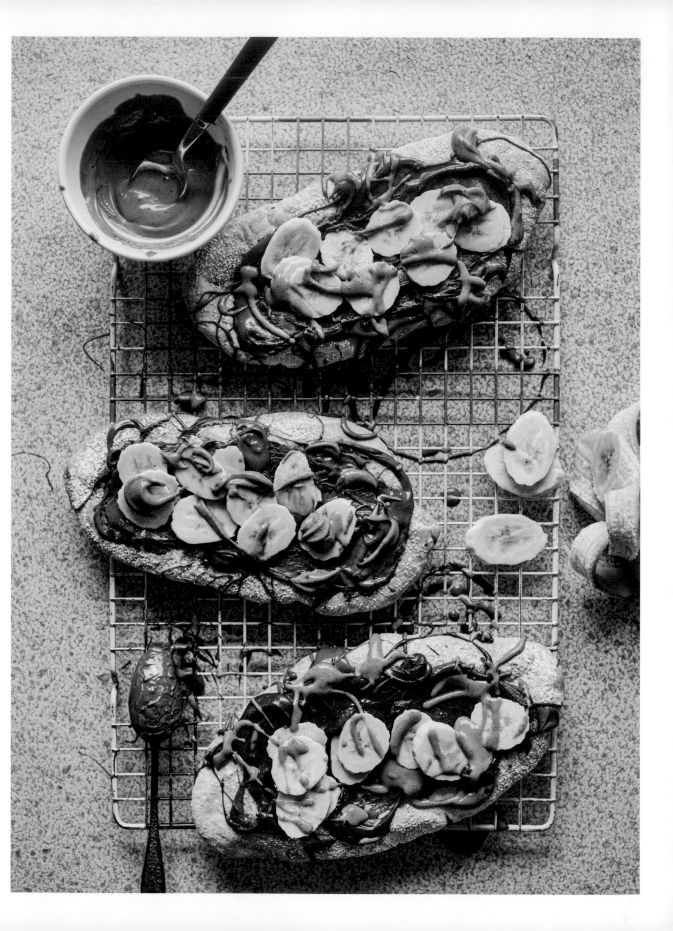

BEAVERTAILS

You're thinking: I can't have those on a diet. We hear you, but indulge us for a moment. These beavertails – baked dough covered in marvellous toppings – are one of our most favourite things.

They remind us of our best holiday – six weeks pootling around Canada. We had our first beavertail atop Grouse Mountain after a morning of terrifying ziplining. Terrifying for us, yes, but imagine being the ashen-faced instructor hoping and praying his clasps, carabiners and public liability insurance would safely carry twenty stone of shrieking Geordie safely across a ravine.

But the beavertails made it all worth it. Try them, love them.

275g (9½oz) self-raising flour
½ tsp salt
1 tsp baking powder
250g (9oz) natural yoghurt
3 tsp icing sugar
65g (2¾oz) milk chocolate chips
2 bananas
2 tbsp smooth peanut butter
2 tbsp milk

Preheat the oven to 200°C fan/425°F/gas mark 7 and place a baking tray in the oven.

In a large bowl, combine the flour, salt and baking powder. Make a well in the middle and pour in the yoghurt. Stir with a fork to combine.

Turn the dough on to a lightly floured surface and knead until it forms a smooth ball. Divide the dough into four and roll each one into a long oblong shape. Take the baking tray from the oven and place the dough strips on it.

Bake for 3–4 minutes, then turn the dough and sprinkle with the icing sugar.

Bake in the oven for 5 more minutes, then remove.

Gently heat the chocolate chips in a microwave until melted (do it in 5–10-second blasts). Spread the melted chocolate over the beavertails.

Slice the bananas and place on top of the chocolate.

Mix the peanut butter with the milk and heat in the microwave for about 10 seconds.

Drizzle the peanut butter over the top of each beavertail, using a spoon.

SMART SWAP

There are loads of different toppings you can try!
Our favourites were the Triple Trip and Bananarama,
which we've combined into this one here. Experiment
with your favourites!

WHOOPSY DAISIES

SERVES: 4
PREP: 5 minutes (plus about 40 minutes setting time)
COOK: 1 minute
CALORIES: 497
DIET: VEG

4 bananas
8 wooden lolly sticks
300g (10½oz) chocolate chips
hundreds and thousands,
    chopped nuts, crushed
    cornflakes (see smart swap)

We're saying nothing as to why these are called whoopsy daisies.

Not one word.

Ssssh. It doesn't need to be said.

;)

Lay some greaseproof paper on a baking sheet.

Cut the bananas in half and gently push each half on to a lolly stick. Place the bananas on the baking sheet and pop into the freezer for 20 minutes.

Gently melt the chocolate in a microwave in 10–20-second blasts, stirring well.

Remove the bananas from the freezer and dip them into the chocolate (you can also spoon it over to cover any bald patches).

Gently roll them in whatever topping you're using and freeze for another 20 minutes.

Serve!

SMART SWAP

These are our favourite toppings, but you can use whatever you like!

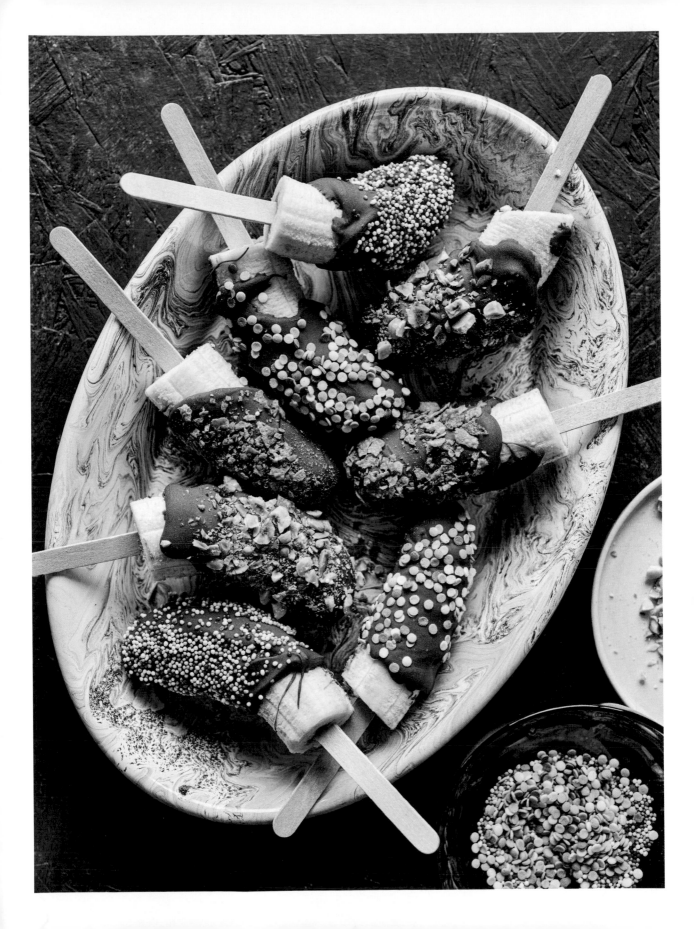

LEMON 'N' LIME BALLS

MAKES: 16 balls
PREP: 10 minutes
(plus 1 hour chilling)
COOK: 0 minutes
CALORIES: 93
DIET: VEG

You might expect me to make a load of testicle-based jokes in an opening about lemon 'n' lime balls, and you know what? You'd be halfway there. These zesty wee buggers are a delight, I promise you, and they're infinitely customizable, but I come not with a recommendation but rather a personal plea!

If you *have* a pair of clackers betwixt your legs, or indeed, if you have easy access to someone who does (I suggest at least being on first name terms before you offer this service), please make sure you're checking them regularly for lumps and bumps. I mention this because I had a scary couple of weeks when I discovered a lump that certainly hadn't been there previously. I'm a hypochondriac at the best of times, but standing in front of the doctor (who was utterly lovely) while he rolled my balls around like the Goblin King from *Labyrinth* wasn't a great time.

My lump went away of its own accord – knowing what a fat bastard I am it was probably a Skittle that had gone on a magical journey – but a mate of Paul's wasn't so lucky. Don't take chances, and don't be shy about getting them out for a second opinion if you need to.

Didn't mean to end on such a sombre note. To compensate, and I apologize wholeheartedly for this, I'll share with you what an ex of mine called them. You'll understand why he's in the past: he called them his jizzberries. Come again? I think not.

175g (6oz) desiccated coconut
250g (9oz) extra-light soft cheese
2 tbsp honey
zest of 1 lime
juice of 1 lemon

Set aside 50g (1¾oz) of the desiccated coconut.

Put the rest of the coconut into a bowl with everything else and whisk well.

Divide the mixture into 14–16 balls and roll them in the reserved coconut.

Place in the fridge for 1 hour to set.

NOTE

Use any flavour combo you like in this – don't be afraid to experiment!

SMART SWAP

If you're not a fan of coconut you could also use crushed Weetabix, for a crispy effect.

SWEETS & TREATS

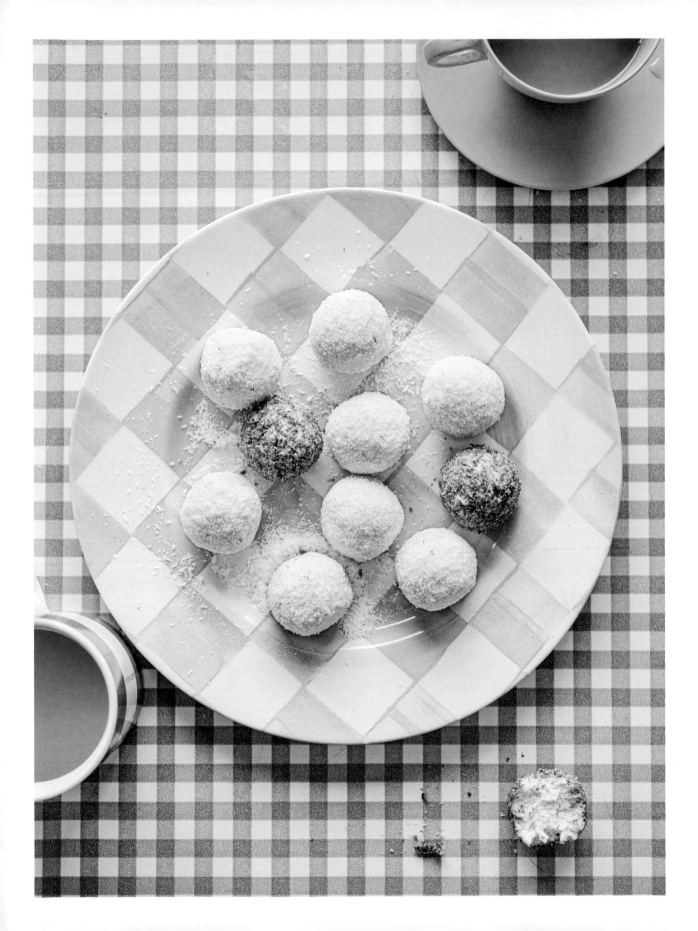

BANOFFEE NICE CREAM

SERVES: 4
PREP: 5 minutes
COOK: 0 minutes
CALORIES: 129
DIET: VEG/GF

Yes, ice cream – but something simple that you can hurl into a blender and pretend to your waiting audience that you've toiled all day stirring and freezing and checking anxiously.

Growing up I quite fancied the idea of being an ice-cream man – driving around dispensing sugary goodness was one thing, but having a van full of ice cream that I could enjoy any time I wanted? Heaven itself. Unfortunately, I don't have the patience to deal with children, nor the self-restraint to not hole myself up in the back and eat everything in sight. They'd find me one day, face down with milk pouring out of my gob, hundreds and thousands and strawberry sauce in my hair.

To the ice cream, then: if you are having trouble finding Werther's Originals, simply accost any elderly relative. If they are anything like my nana used to be, you'll end up with handfuls of them before you've even finished speaking.

4 bananas, sliced and frozen
6 tbsp unsweetened almond milk
8 tsp toffee sauce
4 Werther's Originals, crushed

Place the bananas and almond milk in a food processor and blitz until smooth.

Drizzle 1 teaspoon of toffee sauce into each of four glasses or bowls.

Divide the banana mix among the glasses or bowls, then drizzle over the remaining toffee sauce.

Sprinkle with the Werther's Originals and eat immediately.

NOTE

If this seems a little too runny after blending, you can pop it into the freezer for 10 minutes or so to firm up.

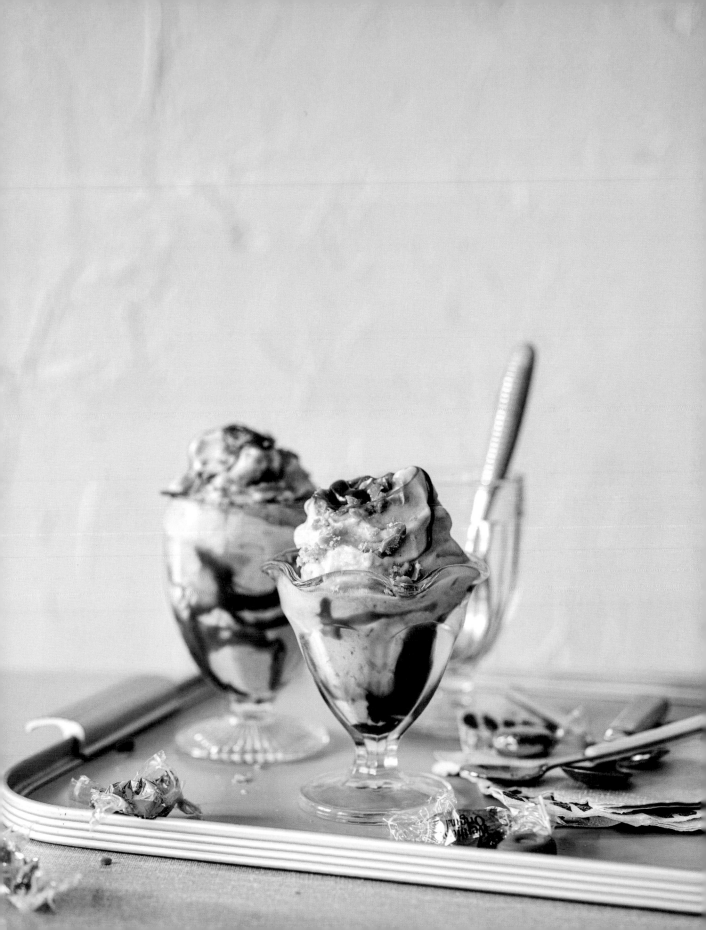

NOT-ELLA DIP

SERVES: 4
PREP: 5 minutes
COOK: 1 minute
CALORIES: 335
DIET: VEG/GF

Isn't Paul clever with that title? Not-Ella! How we laughed at the recipe development bit when he presented that little wonder. Now, come sit down a second.

You may glance at this recipe and blanch at the sight of the chocolate spread, dark chocolate and nuts. Yes, we understand it's a frightening prospect when you're on a diet, but these are really good little desserts, which hit the spot and aren't *too* shocking for your waistline.

The way Paul and I used to diet was to exclude anything like this, with the itch for something forbidden rising and rising until it all got too much and we ended up bingeing on crap for a couple of days. It's a shame cycle: you feel so good sticking to a strict diet, then fall off the wagon because you're depriving yourself, then you feel bloody awful for the next few days. It's a horrendous way of losing weight and it won't last.

Be like us: treat yourself to something delicious at the end of a meal, and you'll get used to enjoying what you have rather than pining for what could be. If your diet says 'no, no, no', look at why that is: no one ever got fat having one decent dessert every now and then.

Goodness: that turned into more of a motivational speech than I expected. My apologies!

100g (3½oz) dark chocolate
100g (3½oz) fat-free crème fraîche
250g (9oz) fat-free Greek yoghurt
4 tbsp honey
2 tbsp chocolate hazelnut spread
2 tsp chopped hazelnuts

Break the chocolate into a bowl and gently warm in the microwave to melt, in 10-second blasts to make sure it doesn't cook.

Gently stir in the crème fraîche, followed by the yoghurt, honey and hazelnut spread.

Divide between four glasses, sprinkle over the hazelnuts and serve.

NOTE

Play around with different flavour combos – our favourites are chocolate and orange, and white chocolate and mint! The base remains the same, just change the chocolate type and the flavourings!

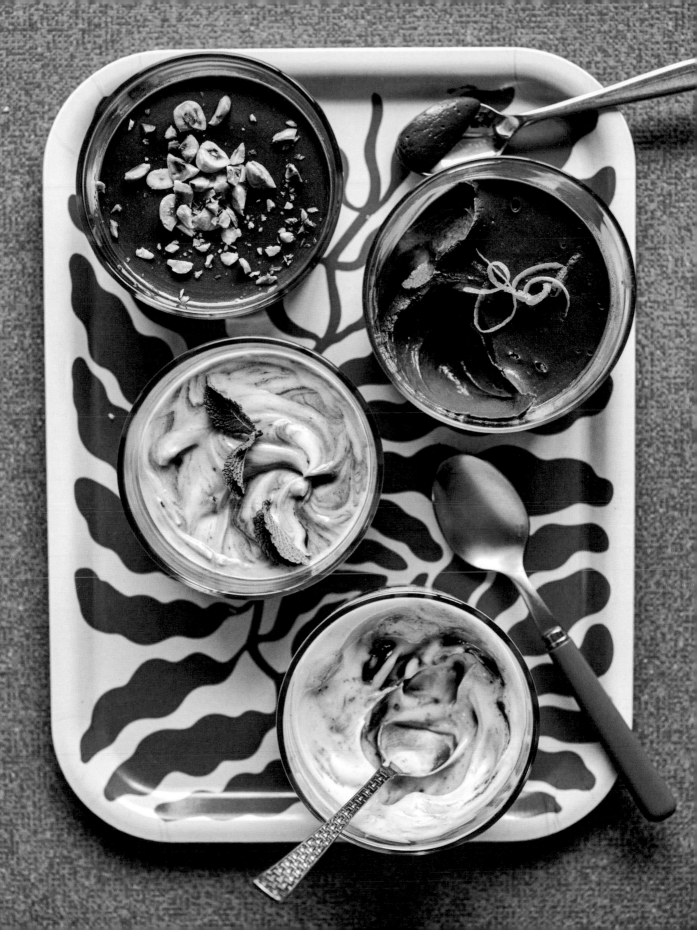

INDEX

Note: page numbers in **bold** refer to photographs.

ACKNOWLEDGEMENTS

JAMES

It's become customary for me to write beautiful words about my beloved Paul at the end of the book, in some beguiling and cunning ploy to make him forget what a terrible husband I am. However, I've already given him some sugar earlier in the book and therefore I'll use this space to tell you one of my favourite anecdotes regarding him. Never miss an opportunity to embarrass the poor sod.

Paul used to be a minute-taker for some very important, can't possibly tell you, people – he would go along to exciting meetings and furiously scribble down everything that was said while desperately trying to stop the eighty-five Biscoff biscuits he had stolen from the refreshments trolley tumbling from his pocket. To assist, the meetings were recorded with audio-sensitive cameras, which automatically moved in response to whoever was speaking. Very high-tech, and Paul does so love a gadget.

Sounds great until Paul drops his pen, nips under the desk to pick it up and accidentally lets out a fart so loud and so booming that all four cameras swivelled around to stare at him accusatorily. Given the gravity of the situation nobody could laugh (and knowing Paul, their noses were probably melting) and so nothing was said, some papers were shuffled and the meeting went on.

He was utterly mortified, poor sod. Still, nobody needs to know …

I do love him, though. He was, is, and shall always be, my perfect other.

I'd also like to extend my thanks to my family who have supported us both during the exciting times and been there to ask why we haven't sent them presents during the difficult ones. You can choose your friends but not your family: we're both damned lucky that mine are really quite good.

I'm told Paul also has a family.

Special thanks to my very best mate Paul 'Blond and Buxom' Hawkins (40), who has successfully completed Year 2 of manning the 'James is in a Tizz' drama hotline.

PAUL

From:	paul.anderson@
Sent:	Friday, May 15, 2020 16:43
To:	james.anderson@
Subject:	Book 2 dedication

Hi – I'm busy trying to work out whether a donkey is just a really small horse. You write something, you love talking about yourself and you're better at the romance things than me

P

PS mention Emma and Danielle or they'll get a cob-on

WIDER THANKS

Paul and I have managed to get the 'sitting down in front of the computer growing steadily fatter' and bashing out recipes routine absolutely nailed. But, without our team, we'd just be two fatty-bum-bums shouting into the internet.

So, a huge thank you to our team: Lauren Whelan (Editorial Director), who has the unfortunate job of listening to our excuses for not hitting deadline (though not this time – boom!), Rebecca Mundy (Publicity Director), who does her best to put us in front of cameras and on the radio, an entirely thankless task when you consider we both look and sound like we're modelled from off-brand Trex. Warm thanks to Grace Paul (Project Editor), whose enthusiasm, vim and vigour know no bounds, even in the face of us cruelly ignoring her messages. Caitriona Horne (Head of Marketing) somehow manages to plod on despite receiving emails from us with the word 'anus' in them, and for that we love her dearly.

Annie Lee (Copy-editor) has turned all our gibberish into proper words and for that we are trooly grateful (never gets old!). Nothing but appreciation for Kay Halsey and Vicky Orchard (Proofreaders) who turned my blistering soft-core erotic novel into a cookbook without raising an eyebrow: amazing job! Our Food Stylists, Photographers, Prop Stylist and Nutritionist (Frankie Unsworth, Sarah Vassallo, Liz and Max Haarala Hamilton, Charlie Phillips and Kerry Torrens respectively) deserve all the credit in the world for turning our plates of dishwater-coloured gruel into the most amazing looking dishes. The people in charge of making this book look so beautiful (Clare Skeats and Diana Talyanina) cannot be thanked enough: I mean, just look at this! It's a cookbook that sings!

Of course, none of this would ever have happened without everyone at Hodder & Stoughton and Yellow Kite. Their support and kindness remain a constant joy.

Thank you to the good, handsome men of Northumberland Fire & Rescue Service – it's not *quite* how I wanted four burly men to come up my back passage, but I'll take it anyway. Call me!

FINALLY

We touched on it at the start of the book but it does so bear repeating. None of this would happen if it wasn't for you. Yes, you. Imagine we're sitting across from you for the full effect of that statement, though honestly we'd probably be texting someone on my phone and paying you lip service. And not that sort of lip service, you dirty bugger.

You bought/borrowed/stole our book. If you didn't do that, we wouldn't be published authors, and all our little mini-dreams would still be in the ether. The support, feedback, compliments and occasional distressing nudes we receive from our Cubs make it all so worthwhile that no amount of fancy thank-you platitudes could ever do it justice.

But please do know how truly grateful we are. We hope you enjoy everything you make, and please do make contact with us on our social media streams. We're pretty good at replying, though that is entirely dependent on whether or not there's something interesting on the TV involving tradesmen.

Good luck with the cooking!

With constant pride and endless love,

JAMES & PAUL x

IF YOU'VE LOVED THE FAST AND FILLING RECIPES
IN THIS BOOK, AND FANCY A FEW MORE LAUGHS,
CHECK OUT OUR FIRST COOKBOOK AND DIET PLANNER:
TWOCHUBBYCUBS: THE COOKBOOK
& TWOCHUBBYCUBS: THE DIET PLANNER

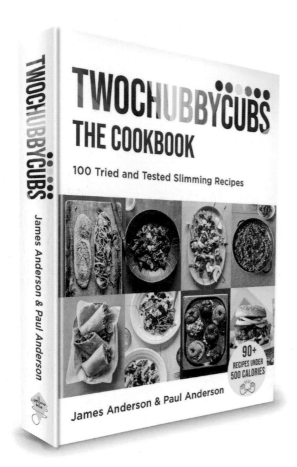

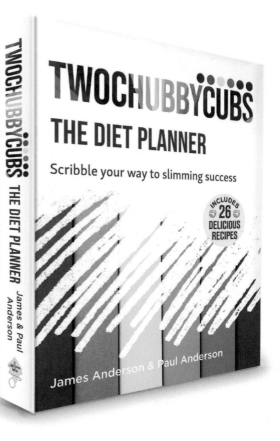

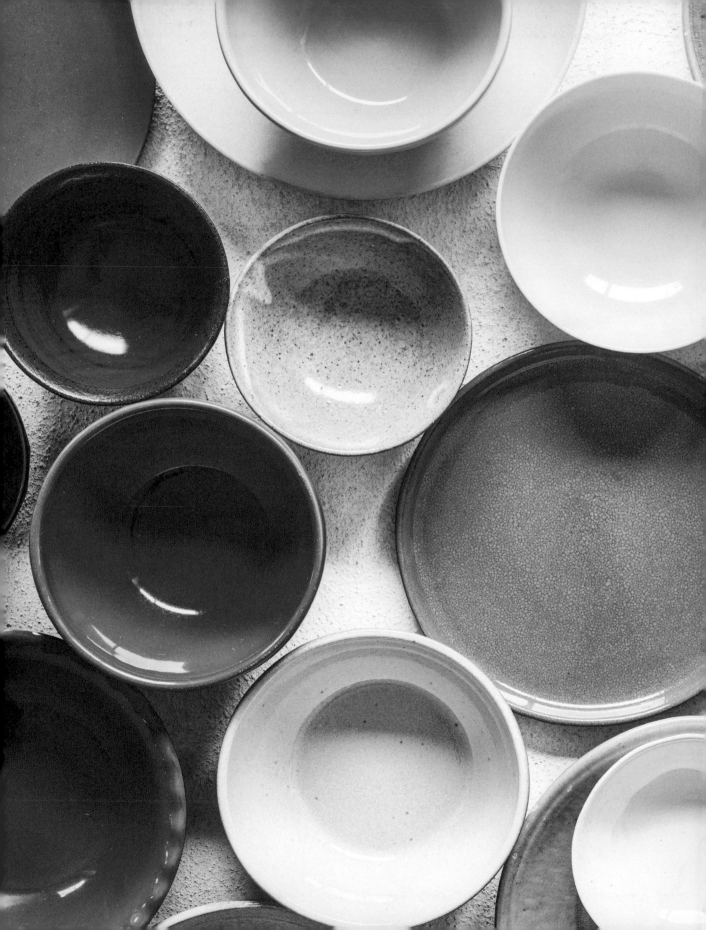